DEPARTMENT OF HEALTH AND SOCIAL SECURITY

DOCTORS TALKING TO PATIENTS

A study of the verbal behaviour
of general practitioners
consulting in their surgeries

PATRICK S. BYRNE
and
BARRIE E. L. LONG

LONDON
HER MAJESTY'S STATIONERY OFFICE

ISBN 0 11 320652 6

CONTENTS

ACKNOWLEDGEMENTS

An incalculable debt is due to more than one hundred GPs who have freely given of their time and advice. This work could not have been completed without their help and interest. As many of these doctors have requested anonymity both for their patients and themselves we cannot publish a list of names.

However, a special thank you must be accorded to Drs C M Harris, G Lloyd and P Freeling for special services. Also to Prof F S Badley and Mr John Lewis for textual assistance and Mr S MacMahon for editorial assistance. Finally to Mrs Martha MacLoughlin who typed patiently.

Needless to say, any errors in the text are the responsibility of the authors.

FOREWORD

This book is the report of a study of the verbal behaviours exhibited by the general practitioner in the consultation—his fundamental work situation. We discovered that the doctors in our study appeared to have achieved set routines of interviewing patients, and that few of them demonstrated the capacity for variations of normal style and performance to meet the needs of those patients whose problems did not fit into an organic disease pattern.

We have attempted to be honest reporters and repeatedly make it clear that the deficiencies revealed in the study are no true fault of the doctor. He is, we say, "both a product and a prisoner of his medical education", which has made no attempt to provide him with behaviours suited to enable him to cope with psycho-social problems. The preponderance of what we term "doctor-centred behaviour" to us stems from the authoritarian teaching and role models which are experienced in hospital, although, even then, not necessarily improperly.

In our contemporary sick society, the psycho-social factors of our patients' illnesses are becoming more frequently observed and demand the use of skills which we have never been formally assisted to acquire. The methods we describe are at present crude and we are in the process of further refining them. We have, however, acquired evidence which suggests that doctors can and will learn new behaviours as long as they see their potential use as relevant to the care of patients. Accordingly we provide some examples and suggest ways of learning in the quest for improved job satisfaction and efficiency in the consultation.

However much we believe in the potential value of our suggested methods, the final arbiters will be our colleagues, the general practitioners. In fact, the methodology proposed may lend itself to practical use by any who have, as a professional requirement, personal interactions with people.

P.S.B.
B.E.L.L.

CHAPTER 1

INTRODUCTION: THE ORIGINS AND ETHICS
OF THE REPORTED STUDY

This research was conceived on the terrace of a house in Westmorland in the summer of 1969. The occasion was marked by the warmth of the evening, food and wine, and the feeling among those present that certain insights had been gained into the behaviour patterns of doctors as a result of some courses for GPs which were, at that time, being conducted in Manchester and Lancaster. What was important was that these insights were quite different from those which formed the "conventional wisdom" of the medical profession and the fact that there was at the time a general paucity of information in the form of literature and research which could help in the development of those insights we had already gained.

The background to the research had been the progressive development of what might be described as a "behavioural science" approach to patient problems which had been central to the development of two courses in behavioural counselling mounted by the Department of General Practice at Manchester in which the staff were P S Byrne, later Professor of General Practice at Manchester, Paul Freeling, a GP and co-author of one of the few books on the consultation, B E L Long, then a Lecturer in Adult Education at Manchester. C M Harris, who left a practice in Liverpool and became a Senior Lecturer in the Department of General Practice, Manchester, also became deeply involved in these courses.

We four had the opportunity at one stage or another to teach and to learn the application of a type of counselling which seeks to modify behaviour in the normal practice requirements of a GP. In the process of working through our teaching programmes we had encountered certain problems which are considered below.

Firstly, we had discovered that those medical people whom we had met, ranging from men who had qualified before the Second World War to students not yet qualified, on the whole showed strong resistance to anything which might be in any way loosely related to a discipline known to them as psychology. To most of them this was something to do with rats and pigeons and had no real relationship with the problems met by a GP in his normal work. One doctor even went so far as to suggest that it was a very apt discipline for a veterinary surgeon but not in any way related to people. This viewpoint for many was substantiated by reference to the content of their various courses in psychology (where these had actually occurred), which had been experiment based and where the bulk of the data was largely derived from studies of animal behaviour.

Secondly, we became aware of a great area of unease surrounding the diagnosis and treatment of the contemporary illnesses classified under the headings of depression, anxiety, neuroses and so forth. This unease became more and more manifest as the various counselling programmes evolved when experienced GPs began to explore therapeutic approaches to these various problems which had nothing to do with chemotherapy.

Thirdly, we became aware, but very slowly, that most doctors seemed to work through a frame of reference which required both patients and illnesses

7

to fit a prejudged pattern. This pattern has a great deal to do with the ways in which doctors learn to cope with the diagnosis of organic illness. Whilst doctors on the whole are expert in the management of organic illness, they are less confident and less equipped to deal with, for example, family problems, or psychosomatic disorder originating in work situations. They had, in fact, few sociological tools of analysis to support their organic diagnostic tools.

Fourthly, we were made aware of the fact that few doctors are able to view the "process" of a consultation in such a way that they are able to make judgements not only about "what they are doing" but also about "how they are doing it". Few doctors, for example, understood the concept of the "dynamic" of a consultation.

Fifthly, we formed the impression that older practitioners had learned habitual patterns of consulting in which even the way they asked questions had become stereotyped. As the "art" of consulting is not taught directly to medical students it seemed likely that each practitioner evolves a pattern of consulting by trial and error which eventually becomes fixed.

Much of our early discussion centred around the possibility of a researcher actually becoming a medical student for six years, because the probability exists that whatever happens to a doctor is most related to his training. This idea would have involved an educationist undergoing the experience of being educated in medicine and would have taken at least eight years to produce anything really valid. Because of the time element, and because of the high risk of the researcher losing any objectivity he might have, this notion was dropped in favour of a shorter term objective look at GPs *in situ*.

The research programme had two aspects. Firstly, there was to be a two-and-a-half-year look at doctors in their surgeries, on their rounds and where possible at the bedside. The purpose of this was to try to discover if there were any features of the consultation which were common to all consultations and whether there were any features of the consultation which could be described as doctor-centred idiosyncrasies. Parallel with this there was to be a scheme of GP trained training which would not only train potential GP trainers but which would also enable the research team to gain insights into the new methods of training which have been developed during the last 20 years.

The second part of the research was to be concerned with the development of totally new learning objectives (largely expressed in behavioural terms) and a parallel development of efficient ways of teaching this new content. The development of the new teaching techniques has been dealt with elsewhere.[1]

The research was promoted by two members of the staff of DH & SS, Drs Wintersgill and Eimerl, who both had experienced some of the new training procedures at Manchester during the period prior to 1971. The internal help and encouragement of these two civil servants gave impetus to those of us who wished to establish the research programme and greatly facilitated the passage of the project through the various committees of the Department itself.

It must now be admitted that in 1971 the project was an act of faith on the part of the DH & SS because there were no possible indicators of success which might have acted as sources of encouragement.

In addition, we have been helped by so many doctors that any list would be inadequate. The staff of the department at Manchester have been supportive and valuable as also have been the many doctors who have attended courses, volunteered tapes, taken part in experiments and indeed acted as guinea-pigs. Altogether some 60 doctors from the United Kingdom have contributed of their time and tapes along with five Dutch doctors and six Irish doctors. In addition some 17 New Zealand doctors and 15 Australian doctors subjected themselves to a variety of tests during 1974, which added considerably to both our research data and teaching methods.

The constraints on the research have been few but they are significant. Ideally there ought to have been a random sample of doctors dealing with a random sample of patients. In fact this is not possible because of the nature of the doctor/patient relationship. We could not force any doctor to contribute to the research any more than we could force a doctor to contribute any of his patients. Consequently, all of the data collected has been volunteered by doctors and all of the patients have been given the choice of being recorded for research purposes or refusing to be recorded. As far as we can gather, not more than about 5 per cent of all patients asked have refused. Consequently, we have an incalculable debt to nearly 2,500 patients.

The tapes contain consultations which may be described as professionally dreadful in terms of the skills or lack of skills shown by doctors and they have contained a very complete range of illnesses met by GPs. The practice of taping complete morning and evening surgeries, with some of our sample five or six times, has produced a relatively random picture of the sort of issues which are treated by a GP. As the research developed, we concentrated more and more upon the surgery situation because that is where the doctor sees the bulk of his patients. We have some tapes of doctors on their rounds but the technical problems of setting up a recorder, and more particularly of establishing a good microphone position, have rendered much of this information useless.

There is one issue which needs to be discussed from the very start. Many researchers claim that the presence of a tape recorder inhibits whatever is going on in the surgery. There is little evidence that this is so. Some of our contributing doctors have claimed that they have made recordings of themselves for our purposes and have subsequently been recorded without their knowledge. They claim there is no perceptible difference in the performance. Equally there is no evidence that patients are inhibited. Many of our helpers tape all their sessions as a matter of course and have a notice in the waiting-room to inform patients of their practice. Some of these patients have discovered they were being taped during the closure of a consultation. They clearly were unaffected by the presence of a recorder during the whole interview, and when they mention the matter to the doctor they also seem unaffected by his statement that the tape is being used exclusively for research purposes.

As to patient behaviour during the interviews, there is no evidence that they have in any way toned down their behaviour because of the recording. A complete range of interviews exists, ranging from a lady wishing to know if the doctor would recommend a Hotpoint or a Tricity electric cooker to a series of the most harrowing interviews dealing with life threatening situations. Whilst we cannot claim for certain that the recording has no effect at all, we can say that our doctors claim it has no effect upon them because they forget the presence of the recorder and microphone and they claim that the recordings sound like perfectly normal patient behaviour.

Another valid point in this respect is the evidence we have about doctor failure.

In a well-edited selection of tapes one would expect editors to try to eliminate their own failure at least to some extent. In fact, with some of our doctors the reverse has happened. They have, and we have been privileged to receive their confidence, insisted upon making special tapes of problem patients as a supplement to their normal tapes. Many of our teaching sessions have been concerned with spectacular failures on the part of the doctor as well as with a series of apparent successes.

The critical issue here is the confidence which has existed between the researchers and the researched. In all cases we have been able to preserve the anonymity of the patients and the professional integrity of the doctors. The one feature which the non-medical researcher has learned is that doctors are expected to work under pressures which do not exist in many other professions. Whilst they do have as a group and individually many shortcomings, these shortcomings are not typical of an entire profession. There are some doctors who do have severe shortcomings in their performance, but there are an equal number of doctors who put far more into their work than any contract with the Health Service or an allegiance to the Hippocratic oath might demand.

The fact, however, remains that this study is a sample of convenience insofar as it is a study of doctors who were prepared to be studied. The only factor which may be weighed against this weakness is the extensive nature of the study. There are recordings of over 2,500 doctor/patient interviews as well as observations of many more.

The part of the study recorded herein was based upon the following methodology. A pilot sample of about 350 consultations volunteered by 15 doctors was analysed in an attempt to discover if there were any consistently observable features in these consultations.

Having erected certain hypotheses, a further selection of 1,000 consultations was analysed from a new set of doctors to check the validity of the hypotheses formulated in the pilot study.

Those defined behaviours which occurred more than five times over the complete sample were listed. A further 500 consultations were analysed to determine the degree to which this list of defined behaviours was capable of describing the majority of behaviours utilised by the doctors in their consultations.

The list of behaviours was then redrawn and attempts were made to categorise the types of behaviour being observed.

The then categorised list was made the subject of a series of experiments in teaching in a variety of settings. A pilot validation of the teaching system was undertaken.

As the research developed various groups of GPs were consulted about the findings and their comments were utilised wherever possible.

In addition, a consultative group of researchers and educationists provided comments from time to time.

Throughout the whole process the staff of the Department of General Practice at Manchester have acted as a reference point and the researcher is greatly indebted to this staff for their help.

CHAPTER 2
DOCTOR BEHAVIOUR IN A CONSULTATION: AN OVERVIEW

There are a number of excellent studies of doctors which refer in one way or another to the doctor/patient consultation. Browne and Freeling in *The Doctor/Patient Relationship*[2] devote a considerable part of their study to the consultation; *The Future General Practitioner*[3] has two lengthy sections and there are literally hundreds of articles and reports which have something to say about the consultation as an act of doctoring. The critical point of most of these studies is that the consultation represents the keystone and the main load of the work of a general practitioner. Paul Freeling once expressed the view that a GP who cannot run an efficient consultation cannot be an efficient GP. To him it is the essence of general practice (*vide* James Spence).[4]

In 1948, Taylor, in his seminal work *Good General Practice*,[5] produced analyses of consultations based upon geographical distinctions of practices, and types of cases, none of which seems to have altered much since that time. There are many ways of examining behaviour, ranging from the complexity of interaction analysis as used by Flanders[6] to the relative simplicity of the "twelve behaviour" system devised by Bales.[7]

The problem with GP behaviour is that it is normally observed in a diadic situation rather than in a small group situation, and also that studies of behaviour in other areas of work have produced categorisations which do not completely fit the doctor/patient situation. The interaction between a group of managers, for example, or that interaction which takes place between teachers and pupils, is derived from a totally different causal base.

The nearest comparable analysis of behaviour is a study by Hays and Larson[8] of interaction between a nurse and a patient which takes place at a hospital bed. This is an interesting study because it concentrates upon the behaviour of the nurse and only refers to the behaviour of the patient where it is necessary to understand the causation of the nurse's behaviour. This technique of analysis proved for us to be fruitful for a variety of reasons.

When studying interaction one is normally concerned with issues like cause and effect. In a study of doctors consulting, as will be seen, much of their behaviour may well be viewed as "cause" and much of patient behaviour as "effect". What is more interesting, however, is the discovery that the patient behaviour rarely appears to become causative. Let us compare two interviews. The first is between a personnel manager and a prospective employee and the second is between a doctor and a patient.

Example 1

PM. "Well, Mr X, I see that you have employment records and references going back over the last ten years. All of them say that you are a very able and diligent manager, and it seems that your employers do not really wish to lose you. Why have you applied to us?"

A. "Well, I believe that we ought to change our jobs every so often so that we do not get stale."

P. "That's an interesting idea—what do you mean by 'getting stale'?"

11

A. "Well, all jobs are made up of some routine and some challenge. As time goes on the challenge in any line job becomes less and less. When that happens either the job gets dull or the manager does."

P. "Do you think that many managers get dulled by their jobs?"

A. "On the whole, yes, unless you keep on getting promotion. In small companies promotion is difficult so it is often worth making a sideways move."

P. "This job, then, is a sideways move for you?"

A. "Yes, on the face of it there is little increase in salary and not much more in the way of responsibility."

P. "Do you mean that you respond well to responsibility?"

A. "That's what real management is all about. If a job has no responsibility it means that there is no real management activity. It also means, in small organisations, that owners do not trust their employees."

P. "Is your experience in small organisations leading you to the conclusion that most owners do not trust employees?"

A. "Yes. On the whole I see owners rushing around doing jobs that are better done by their employees. I don't know what makes them do it, but it seems they are quite unable to stop themselves. It has a very bad effect upon workers, who resent their bosses doing the jobs they are paid to do."

P. "How then should bosses treat workers?"

A. "If a man is employed to do a job he should be paid a fair wage and he should be given the chance to show that he can do that job and more without his boss breathing down his neck."

In this interview, the personnel manager initiates the discussion and is thus causative, but all of his subsequent questions are the result of something the interviewee has previously said. Thus all of his interventions are really effects rather than causes.

Example 2

D. "Well now, here you are again. How are things?"

P. "Oh, doctor, I have not been taking all those pills you gave me. They didn't seem to agree with me."

D. "Ah ha. Have you been getting in your exercise every day?"

P. "Oh, yes, doctor. Every morning I walk to work and I walk home at night. That's nearly four miles a day."

D. "Mmm. Now then, how about that leg?"

P. "Oh, that's much better now. The scar is still there though. I expect it will go in time."

D. "How about the wife. Is she getting about all right?"

P. "Yes. She gets out of a morning and goes down to the shops. She takes the bus down to the station, you know, and walks from there."

D. "You're sleeping all right, aren't you?"

P. "Well, I still take those tablets, doctor."

D. "Good. Well now. Take this to Mr Green and get it made up. There are some different pills. Different colour, you know. Let me know how things are getting on. Don't forget your umbrella. 'Bye-bye."

In this interview all of the patient's replies to questions have been absorbed by the doctor who has never used any of the information given to develop further responses. It is clear that he is reacting to the information about the

12

pills, but he does not bother to investigate what happened to the patient when he took the pills. The example is perhaps an extreme case of what is indeed a simple "repeat prescription". What is important, however, is that the doctor provides all of the causes and the patient all of the effects. In our recorded consultations this relationship describes more than 75 per cent of what took place. Not more than one consultation in 20 would resemble Example 1.

This cause and effect pattern means that it is possible to apply the Hayes and Larsen technique to the doctor/patient consultation and to be able to deal with the largest part of the doctor's behaviour without reference to any patient-caused behaviour. Those parts of a doctor's behaviour which are reactive should then become separate studies. We have not undertaken a study of patient behaviour.

With reference to Example 2 above, let us examine all of the patient's responses and offer an interpretation.

Response 1 The patient informs the doctor that he has not been following his prescribed medication programme. He then produces a vague reason for not doing so. The doctor does not, however, respond to this.

Response 2 Here the patient feels he has done what was required and might well be seeking some praise. The doctor does not appear to give it.

Response 3 This time the patient is probably looking for some sort of reassurance. If he was, then he was unlucky.

Response 4 It is possible that the patient is still looking for some sort of reassurance that his wife is following her prescribed and correct treatment.

Response 5 This response caused the doctor concerned the greatest concern when he heard the tape. At the time he felt it was confirmation that the patient was sleeping. In fact, it was a clear piece of evasion and possibly a belated attempt to provoke some sort of response in the doctor. All it produced, however, was the end of the consultation.

Now we can analyse the doctor. He starts with a recognition of the patient which, incidentally, is quite different from his standard opening which is, "Hello, and what can we do for you today?" or for young women, "Hello, and what can we do *you* for today?" Then he asks a broad question. His next noise, "Ah ha," indicates that he has understood what the patient has said. He then asks a question which narrows the patient down to a specific reply.

His third intervention, "Mmm," again indicates he has heard the patient's response and it is followed by a quite specific question.

The fourth intervention changes the subject completely by his broad question, "How about the wife?" but this is promptly narrowed down to a nearly closed question about her ability to get about.

The fifth intervention might charitably be seen as a very probing question, but in fact it serves as nothing of the sort because the patient's response is nil.

Finally, the doctor does a number of things in a given sequence. "Good. Well now." This indicates that the enquiry is over and something else is about to start. Then follows a clear instruction. Then he offers a little supplementary information to indicate that he has noted the patient's earlier statement about the pills. "Different colour, you know," however, is a subtle piece of self-

13

justification. "Let me know how things are getting on" indicates that the consultation is now terminated and the next statement, "Don't forget your umbrella," finally closes off any chance the patient may have had to reply.

This particular consultation has been discussed in depth with the doctor concerned, who claimed that this particular patient required simply a repeat prescription and he felt that he had to go through the formalities. The consultation was also at the end of a very busy surgery which happened to coincide with an outbreak of influenza. Consequently the surgery was full and he was about to go off on twice his normal number of visits. The patient was a regular attender, working far beyond retirement age. He had just had a number of varicose veins removed from his leg. The doctor also claimed that he felt forced to keep this patient under tight rein for otherwise he would talk for hours. This claim, however, could not be substantiated from other of this doctor's consultations, which were all short and made up of largely closed questions in which the patient was likely to answer "Yes" or "No". His style of consulting was highly mechanistic.

Here is an extreme example of a doctor who works through a rigid frame of reference. *The Future General Practitioner*[3] contains the following statement:

"The doctor may insist on focusing on certain aspects of the patient's problem because they are the easiest for him to handle. He will then refuse to allow the patient to tell him anything else, or refuse to hear. To obtain his greatest satisfaction the doctor usually wants to find a patient with a serious, acute illness that has interesting features—elicited and recognised by him with great acumen—and one who responds rapidly, completely and gratefully to proper therapy."

That statement was written by a group of doctors about doctors and is another way of describing a narrow frame of reference. If the doctor has a perception of illness which is conditioned by a predisposition towards clear-cut diagnosis and rapid efficacious curative procedures, he is not going to respond well to vague offers of self by the patient. It is also unlikely that he will be wholly at ease when coping with emotional problems which on the whole do not lend themselves to clear-cut diagnoses nor to rapid cures.

Yet it is true to say that most general practitioners display to some extent this preference in their practice of medicine. There must be some reason for this. Although our evidence is incomplete, it is apparent that British GPs do see, on average, about 10 patients more per day than their Dutch, Australian or New Zealand counterparts. Consequently the amount of time available for each patient will be less and consultations may contain less exploration of vague emotional areas. More important perhaps, however, is the predisposition towards organic medicine which is still a feature of medical education and hence a conditioned factor of GPs' thinking.

A prime purpose of the doctor is to provide a system of patient protection against disease, and consequently, quite rightly, the basic training of a doctor still emphasises the body systems, ie organic disease. It would be improper to advocate a complete reorganisation of medical education on the supposed basis of a massive increase in psychosomatic disorder, because at this moment we simply do not know what proportion of a doctor's work is purely organic and what proportion is purely psychological and/or psychosomatic. Estimates vary widely, from 80 per cent to 5 per cent, and until objectively based figures are

14

produced no real reappraisal of medical education can be rational.

Perhaps more significant is a point made in 1960 by Scott, Anderson and Cartwright.[9] They divide a doctor's therapeutic behaviour into four categories: advice, explanation, discussion and listening. There has always been considerable evidence in the field of communication studies that most listening is selective, while there is no evidence that doctors are any less selective than are any other group. The paper referred to considers listening to be a valuable part of the doctor's skill pattern. There is little evidence that "listening" as such appears to be an integral part of medical training, and if it is taught it is always as a function of something else. As many other professional groups now find it necessary to emphasise listening skills in their own development, there might well be a message here for medical educators. In Example 2 (above) there is considerable evidence that the doctor either did not hear what the patient was saying, or that he chose to select out of what was said that which he wished to hear.

There is, of course, another side to the coin. There are doctors who can and do conduct skilful analyses of emotional problems and who display skills which psychotherapists would applaud. In *Learning to Care*, Byrne and Long[10] quote the following case as an example of a totally different type of consultation. It is unashamedly included here as an example of what a GP may do with a rather different frame of reference.

(The authors are indebted to Dr C M Harris for providing this material.[10])

D. "Come in. . . . Good morning. . . . Sorry to keep you waiting, Mrs M——. These are two medical students."
P. "I presumed so."
D. "That's okay?"
P. "Yes."
D. "Please sit down."
P. "After seven children I've seen a lot of them."
D. "A lot of medical students?"
P. "Yes."
D. "So what can I do for you?"

Up to this point Mrs M—— has been bright and has enveloped some of her responses in laughter, especially the one concerning the number of medical students she has seen.

P. "To be quite honest I don't know. I just feel awful. I keep going hot and cold. My eyes come up. I'm nearly forty-five and I suppose I must be on the change now?"
D. "What shall I tell you now?"
P. (Laughter) "No. . . . Women have done it before."
D. "Is that what you are telling yourself?"
P. "That's what I'm presuming. . . . I don't know."
D. "Mmm, Mmm" (agreement noises). "What does the change mean to you?"
P. "I don't know. But my periods are some months heavy . . . some months I have two."
D. "Mmm, Mmm."
P. "Last month I had two and the one now was due last Friday."

15

D. "Mmm, Mmm. What does the change mean as an idea to you? I mean. . . ."

P. "Well, I don't know. I have an idea that it is usual for women. They have these hot flushes, and they don't feel for this and they don't feel for that . . . but my mother used to have blackouts."

D. "When she was on the change, you mean?"

P. "Yes."

D. "Mmm. And you are worried you would be. . . ."

P. "Well, I don't know . . . but I'm frightened."

D. "Mmm, Mmm. Frightened of what?"

P. "Of getting blackouts, or anything like that." (Voice level drops.)

D. "You are frightened of more than blackouts?"

P. (Nervous laugh) "Well, it's not that I choose to. We used to find her miles away on buses."

Short silence. Mrs M—— has started to cry.

D. "Go on."

P. (Crying openly) "Well, she never knew how she got there."

D. "Mmm, Mmm. And that was supposed to be due to the change?"

P. "Well, that's what she told me. I don't know."

D. "And when did she tell you that?"

P. (Continues crying for a few seconds) "Well, it's years ago. She's dead now. I think she was going out of her mind. Well, it's years ago . . . twenty-three years ago."

D. "Mmm, Mmm."

P. "Well, she used to go out on the bus. Then they'd find her miles away. And she never knew how. I never knew, but my father used to say she was 'on the change'."

D. "So for the last twenty years you have thought of the change as a time when you . . . ?"

P. "Well, I have really."

D. "So, when you get to forty-five and your periods get irregular. . . ."

P. "Well, you think. Well, you do get worried . . . I suppose. I don't know."

D. "But you know, because you've seen in the past twenty years other women get past the age of change without going the way your mother went? So does that mean you feel more like her than . . . ?"

P. "Well, you know, are these things inherited—that's what I want to know? That's what worried me."

D. "Did she keep on doing it for years, or was it just for a short space in time?"

P. "Well, no. I think it went on for a couple of years, and then she used to have these blackouts . . . and she used to haemorrhage from the nose."

D. "Mmm."

P. "And she used to go unconscious. And she had a baby when she was forty-one. And I remember them saying at the time that she would probably be all right then. But as far as I remember she was worse."

D. "After having the baby?"

P. "Yes."

D. "Well, do you feel that these things which happened to her were connected with having a baby at forty-one?"

P. "Well, I don't know. People say that if you have a baby on the turn then you are all right."

16

D. "What kind of treatment did she have when she was doing this?"

P. "Well, she didn't really. She was old-fashioned. She wouldn't go anywhere. She wouldn't go to the doctor, and she wouldn't go to the hospital. She did eventually. We insisted, and they found nothing wrong with her. She had . . . what did she have . . . this brain test?"

D. "An EEG?"

P. "Mmm, Mmm. She had that and they didn't find anything. She was very heavy and they said she had to cut her weight down, but she didn't."

D. "Mmm, Mmm."

P. "But she just carried on and then she just died suddenly. She was fifty-nine. . . . Of heart failure and bronchitis."

D. "Is that on your mind as well?"

P. "No, not really. I don't think about that. It's just that I think about this . . . um, um . . . change. God help I don't go like her."

D. "Do you have any sisters?"

P. "Mmm, Mmm."

D. "Are they older than you or younger?"

P. "They are younger."

D. "Have they got the same kind of fears about the change as you?"

P. "I don't know. I've never asked them. One's twenty-eight, and the other's thirty-six."

D. "So you are a good bit older than them?"

P. "Yes. I can remember, they can't."

D. "There perhaps was a time when you were almost as much their mother as your mother was?"

P. "Well, it could be. Well, I almost brought the others up, you know."

D. "Are you a motherly person?"

P. "Well, I've got seven of my own." (She has stopped crying and is now beginning to laugh again.) "So I am. . . . Yes."

D. "Have you talked to anybody or your husband about this yet?"

P. "No, I haven't."

D. "So you've bottled it all up. And now it just won't stay bottled any more."

P. (Crying again) "No, but it's silly. . . . Nobody ever asked me before, before you asked me. And I know it's there when I think about it."

D. "When you came here today had you intended to tell me this?"

P. "No."

D. "How come you did tell me then?"

P. "I suppose I didn't try really . . . you don't." (Crying again) "I don't know. It's something you don't talk about. If you did someone would say you were daft. I suppose it's inside you really. I've had a very happy life, my mother didn't. Fair enough. Whether that had anything to do with it, I don't know."

D. "You have had a happy married life?"

P. "Well, I have done. My mother didn't. My father used to knock her about. The usual story, you know. Whether that had anything to do with it I don't know."

D. "Why do you think your husband would think you were daft if you were to tell him?"

P. "Well, he's very sensible. He says these things don't happen and he'd go on as though it were all right. I don't know. I'm just saying this."

17

D. "But if he could see how important it was to you . . . do you think he would react like that?"

P. "Well, if he knew how important it was . . . well . . . well . . . it was him who made me come here. He said, 'Why don't you go and see the doctor, you keep putting it off and putting it off, and saying it's the change, it could be anything'." (Mrs M—— still showing signs of distress.)

D. "Do you feel any different now, from when you came in?"

P. "I don't know. It's a silly thing. You have seven children and you do this and you do that. You've got to get it behind yourself. You pretend it's not there, but it's there all the time. And you keep thinking to yourself, well, it might be all right. I've been happily married, why worry?"

D. "So today you've done something very different from what you normally do?"

P. "I have, yes. I never expected it."

D. "Right. I think that's very good. I'd like you to come back and see me next week."

P. (Still crying) "Is it the change?"

D. "If your periods have been going irregular then it may be. Sure."

P. "Well, I've always been regular, let's face it . . . as far as these things go. Now it goes that I have none this month and then next month I have two."

D. "Okay. We can go into those sort of details next week. But I think you've done something very big this week. I don't want to start confusing you now with all sorts of little details."

This consultation on audio-tape has been played to a large number of GP teacher groups as an example of a teaching situation. Their response, however, has usually been at the level of organic medicine. The doctor, C M Harris, has invariably been asked to justify his not having conducted a whole series of tests upon this woman to determine whether or not she was menopausal, pregnant or whatever. He has also been asked to justify why he did not indulge himself, or the patient, in an extensive prescriptive process. He has consistently taken the view that this consultation is complete and only requires the patient to go away and think. He has caused her to verbalise a whole range of fears and confront issues and to him that is enough. Curiously (or perhaps not) the GP who provided Example 2 felt that he ought to have prescribed an anti-depressant.

This book then is concerned largely with the sorts of issues which have been talked about here. It is largely a pilot study of the behaviours of doctors seen in their surgeries, but it attempts to analyse these behaviours not in medical but in social terms. It will not attempt to provide more sets of data to be crunched in computers unless those sets of data are vital to the theme. Its purpose, as far as it is possible, is to provide a non-judgemental view of how doctors behave, in the hope that it will cause discussion between interested groups who will be responsible for those developments which we hope it may effect.

CHAPTER 3

THE STRUCTURE OF THE CONSULTATION: AN ANALYSIS OF BEHAVIOURAL PHASES

The first task undertaken by the researcher was to listen to a large number of consultations to discover what sorts of behavioural phenomena were occurring. There is, of course, a standard medical model of the consultation which describes in medical terms what should happen. It follows the procedure below:

1 History taking.
2 Examination.
3 Diagnosis.
4 Treatment.

This description tells us what is happening in terms of the medical procedures which are being followed, but it does not tell us much about what sort of process is going on between the two or more persons involved. If we examine two similar interpretations of counselling, we might be able to observe the type of distinctions which are critical to our methods of analysis.

Counselling, as a goal-seeking activity, follows a number of logical steps which are similar to most decision-making models:

1 Collect and collate data relevant to felt needs.
2 From data define problem(s).
3 Generate possible solutions to problem(s).
4 Examine implications of solutions.
5 Select a solution or solutions.
6 Implement a solution.
7 Evaluate the results.

This is a description of the required logical steps of counselling but not a description of the process of what takes place between the counsellor and the counsellee during counselling. Another way of expressing this process might be as follows (from the standpoint of the counsellor):

1 Relate to the client (counsellee).
2 Enable the client to talk about his problems.
3 Utilising such skills as reflecting, interpreting and silence, enable the client to probe deeply into causation so that he understands his problem.
4 Allow the client to define his own problem.
5 Enable the client to generate his own solutions to his own problem, utilising the same skills as in (3) above.
6 Taking each solution in turn, examine the degree to which the client feels he is able to appreciate the consequences of each of his solutions. (Utilising the client's own words and ideas, the counsellor may at this stage choose to confront the client with any inconsistencies in his approach to his problem.)
7 If the client so wishes, enable him to select one or more of his own solutions to his own problem and then enable the client to terminate the interview.
8 Counsellors do not get involved in enabling clients to implement solutions.

What we have done here is to clothe the first rather sterile decision-making model with a description of some of the behaviours of a counsellor, and thus by implication we are to a large extent predicting the behaviour of the client. This is far from a complete description of what happens in counselling, but it does have the virtue of providing us with some insights into the nature of this rather specialised form of communication.

When doctors talk to patients various descriptions may be referred to which attempt to describe, in non-medical terms, what is happening. Browne and Freeling indicate[2] that various psychoanalytic models may be used and also feel that Eric Bernes' [11] transactional analysis might well describe the activity. Certainly Eric Bernes' "game" approach does describe a whole range of human interactions in a spectacular way. To a large extent this approach is helpful in describing the overall picture of what is happening between doctors and patients.

Michael Balint, in his book *The Doctor, his Patients and the Illness*,[12] has an excellent section on what he describes as "The Apostolic Function", in which he argues that doctors have virtually conditioned patients to behave in a certain way. This was summed up by a splendid New Zealand GP who said: "In order to have the privilege of talking to your doctor, you need to fulfil the essential precondition of being sick. Then you may go to him and ask him if he will perform his professional services upon you." Most doctors seem to agree that Balint was correct and admit that what the patients may offer is often not related to the reason for their attendance. When this does happen in consultations, one may observe an interesting game being played by the patient and sometimes also by the doctor. Patients may make offers which are concealed in answers to questions, such as the reply in Example 2 in the previous chapter: "Oh, doctor, I've not been taking those pills. They didn't seem to agree with me."

This is not the same as saying: "I am not taking those pills."

The most famous of all patient tricks is, of course, the Parthian shot of: "Oh, by the way, doctor. . . ." Almost inevitably this happens towards the end of a consultation and is not necessarily preceded by any intimation that the patient wanted to say something other than what has been said. Most doctors agree that when they hear those words they start to suffer unpleasant feelings in various parts of their anatomy which have no clear organic cause.

One interesting theory which might describe patient behaviour is the "balloon theory". This likens the initial relationship between two people to a military situation with two armies well dug into their trenches on Christmas morning. Neither side wishes to have a shooting match that day but each is unaware of the intentions and feelings of the other. One side then raises a small balloon just above the level of the parapet. If it is shot down the intentions of the other party are clear. If, however, the enemy reciprocates by raising another small balloon then a new game is being played. The first army proceeds to hoist a larger balloon rather higher than its first. The second army then reciprocates. The game finally goes on until one side or the other feels confident enough actually to get up on to the parapet and wave to the other side.

The same process may take place between two human beings who go through a series of manoeuvres to discover whether or not the other party is prepared to listen to what they really want to say. The shooting down of the balloon at any stage usually indicates that there is not a relationship of confidence between the two parties and nothing of moment will be said.

The problem to which this research addressed itself was simple. We were seeking to discover what patterns of behaviour doctors appeared to follow in their consulting rooms and the degree to which the patterns were repetitive among doctors.

One of our great problems was to pin down a sequence which could be seen to occur frequently. The real difficulty was not defining the events but sequencing them in a logical form. The logical form finally agreed rarely appears in practice and should be seen as an ideal. As we shall see, there are a variety of reasons for this. The logical sequence of events we discovered to be as follows:

I   The doctor establishes a relationship with the patient.

II   The doctor either attempts to discover or actually discovers the reason for the patient's attendance.

III The doctor conducts a verbal or physical examination or both.

IV The doctor, or the doctor and the patient, or the patient (in that order of probability) consider the condition.

V   The doctor, and occasionally the patient, detail treatment or further investigation.

VI The consultation is terminated usually by the doctor.

I Relating to the patient

Normally relating to the patient takes very little time. It is usually contained in a few words such as: "Hello, Mr X, what can I do for you today?" All that has happened here is that the doctor has shown that he recognises the patient and is straight into phase two, "discovering the reason for attendance". Most doctors use the same form of words for most of their patients.

An occasion when this short stage might take more time is when a new patient arrives. The doctor will require information for his records which he might see as wholly part of his clerical function. The new patient, however, might well view it as something else. Take the following example:

D. "Good morning. I am Dr Smith. You are a new patient, aren't you, Mrs A——? Now then, how long have you lived here?"

P. "Oh, we only moved in a week ago."

D. "Oh, that's nice, where to?"

P. "We bought a bungalow up on the new estate. Do you know the area?"

D. "Up beyond Mountsandel Road. Oh, yes. They are nice. And you're married?"

P. "Yes, and two children. Girl and boy, six and two."

D. "That's well planned. What are their names?"

P. "Fenella and Graham. After my parents, you know."

D. "That's good. And how old are you?"

P. "Me? Oh, I'm twenty-nine, going on thirty."

D. "Splendid. Well now. There are a few other bits of information I will need but we can forget that for now. What is it that has brought you here?"

It may well be that the doctor was only following a set routine, but he was able to use the time to gain a lot of personal information about his new patient, and performed in a manner which was friendly and open, thus offering the opening for a good doctor/patient relationship.

This particular doctor also resisted the temptation to which some are prone of launching himself into an immediate statement about the rules and regulations of his practice. These constraints on patient behaviour, however, came out as the consultation progressed. An example is as follows:

Mrs A—— mentioned that her son had symptoms which sounded like a possible asthmatic condition. Because of the weather she had not brought him to the surgery. The doctor took this information and made this comment:

"Well now, I don't like the sound of that. I'll pop in this afternoon and we'll have a look. After surgery I get a quick bite of lunch, then I go out on call from about 1.30 to 3.30. We have another surgery from 4.15 to 6.30 and the first hour and a half are appointments only. If you want me when I'm on call just ring here and they will get in touch with me."

There does not seem to be much evidence that there is any wide range of relating behaviours. Most GPs demonstrate a fairly standard routine form of words which cover most patients. It is only when the patient is new or when a third party is present that any significant variation in words occurs. The GPs covered in this research demonstrated that they use not more than three forms of words to cover most of their situations. The only changes which have been observed are related to the time at which a patient enters the consulting room and the number of patients who have preceded that patient. A doctor who starts the day with something like, "Hello. Good morning, Mr X, and how are you today?" may well become, "Hello. What is it then?" by the end of a long evening surgery. Unless a doctor is dealing with a new patient (and even then not always) relating usually only takes up a few seconds of time, not more than 10 or 15 being the norm.

II Discovering the reason for the patient's attendance

Unlike "relating", which is found in all consultations, discovering the reason for attendance may not be so apparent. There are a variety of situations, eg "progress cases" (see Taylor), in which the reason for the attendance may well have been considered at a previous consultation. For ante-natal clinics, post-natal clinics, returning referrals and most patients wishing repeat prescriptions who actually get into the consulting room, the doctor appears to have a pre-determined agenda.

What is much more interesting about this particular activity is how long it lasts after the doctor has given the signal that it may begin. The signal usually takes the form of what we will later describe as a "Broad opening", eg "And what can we do for you today?" or "What brings you here today?" or even "How are you today?" What is significant is what the doctor says and does after the patient replies to this particular opening.

Take the following patient statement, which occurs very frequently in one form or another: "Well, I'm feeling run down. I've got a pain in my back and I just feel tired all day."

The following are a selection of the responses which have been recorded:

"Mmm. Right, just go into the next room and get undressed. I'll be along in a minute."

"Tell me. Just where is this pain?"

"When do you feel tired? In the morning when you get up or in the afternoon?"

"Do you have headaches and pains behind the eyes?"

"I think you're depressed. How do you feel about that?"

22

"What sort of pain is it?"

"What do you mean by 'I feel tired all day'?"

"Yes, go on."

"You look very pale."

Here are nine responses to the same input. They range from a response in which the doctor has already made up his mind and is preparing to consider a treatment, to a doctor who is preparing for a long discussion about further patient-perceived symptoms. Also discernible is the instant organic approach in which the doctor is preparing to work at a physical, before any further verbal, examination.

To some extent the doctor can be assisted by patients who will present him with a clear description of a set of symptoms. For example, during an influenza epidemic one doctor produced a tape in which five patients consecutively appeared with almost identical speeches:

"Well, doctor, as you can see, I've got a bad cold, I've got a headache, little appetite and pains in the muscles, here."

This particular doctor was not an instant prescriber and used the tape to show the dangers of accepting all this information as routine. Out of the fifth and last patient he also got, after two or three questions, the fact that he had some very badly swollen glands and discovered that this patient was not suffering from influenza.

GPs also suffer problems with recent immigrants who have only a bare command of the language (if any at all) and who occasionally present themselves in surgery with alleged interpreters who have little more ability to communicate than has the patient. There is one amusing episode in which three persons turned up and after five minutes' confusion the interpreter finally announced to the doctor the fact that:

"He says his wife is not well and would you be so kind as to examine her because he says he is all right today apart from a pain in his hand which he does not want to talk to you about today if you please. Thank you."

As will be noted from the subsequent chapter on dysfunction, the quantity of time spent on Phase II ranges from no time at all to over eight minutes.

A number of variables appear to influence the time a doctor elects to spend on Phase II.

(a) The degree to which a doctor is prepared to accept the first thing a patient may say.

(b) The degree of clarity with which the patient presents his symptoms.

(c) The number of patients who have actually preceded the patient in question and the number still waiting outside.

(d) The degree to which the doctor is oriented towards organic illness.

(e) The doctor's beliefs about himself and about his patients.

III Conducting a verbal or physical examination or both

This phase(s) of a consultation may also not appear. Taylor again defines one group of consultations as "quickies". These might be requests for one or more of the various bits of paper doctors issue. Many repeat prescriptions and a considerable amount of family planning activity seems not to have any associated examination. Patients returning after a referral to hospital also do not often undergo further examination. Furthermore, while many doctors

23

seemed to get involved in moral or ethical debates when dealing with certain family planning requests, more did so when dealing with requests for abortion.

In 73 per cent of the consultations studies there was some physical or verbal examination. Depending upon how well the doctor has understood why the patient is present the examination may last from a few seconds to many minutes. A fairly short example may be seen in this management of a repeat prescription.

"Hello, Mr J——. Back for your prescription? Yes. Good. Now then, tell me, when you take these tablets do you feel all right afterwards?"

"Well, yes, doctor."

"No strange pains or dizziness?"

"Not a thing, doc. No problems at all. All systems go."

"That's fine. All I wanted to know. Okay. Here you are then. See you in a month. Okay? Cheerio."

Verbal and physical examinations are not necessarily separate activities. Many doctors perform both together. The following extract is taken from a consultation in which the patient has complained about chest pain and the doctor quickly had him stripped to the waist.

D. "Right now, breathe in, will you? Good. Again. Good. Tell me, when do you get these pains?"

P. "Not all the time, doc. Some days I very often don't get them at all."

D. "Deep breath, please. Good. And again, please. How many cigarettes do you smoke a day?"

P. "Oh. I gave it up last week."

D. "Breathe. Good. Yes. Well, before you gave it up, how many?"

P. "Oh, twenty, sometimes thirty."

D. "Mmm. Yes. Well, there is certainly some obstruction here. Let's have a listen to your tubes again. Breathe. Good. Do you get short of breath when you do anything energetic?"

P. "Like what?"

D. "Well. Running upstairs."

P. "Well, I don't run upstairs now."

D. "Why not?"

P. "Well, I'm afraid it might come on."

D. "Breathe. Right. Now then, I want you to blow into this thing. It'll tell me how much puff you've got."

P. "In there?"

D. "Yes, in there."

   Patient blows.

D. "Tell me, what do you do at work?"

P. "I drive a loader."

D. "Is it hard work?"

P. "Only when they don't load the sacks proper. Then I have to pick them up and reload them."

D. "What do these sacks weigh?"

P. "Most times about a hundredweight."

Few doctors actually explain what they are doing when they examine patients physically, so much so that it is surprising to find a doctor who does keep up a running commentary on his work.

D. "Now then, this is a stethoscope. With it I can hear your heart and the air passing into your lungs. It might be a touch cold. Now then, deep breath. Good. I'm listening to your heartbeat now. Now then, deep breath. Now I'm listening to your lungs. They sound clear. Good. Another, please."

P. "What are you doing now?"

D. "Well, your lungs and heart aren't only around the fourth rib, you know. They come down here as well."

Although this particular excerpt took place with an adult it is more common with children. A few doctors appear to use the technique to reassure children whilst they are being examined.

IV Consideration of patient condition

Of all the six phases in a consultation, this one is the only one which may be clearly marked as "optional under all circumstances". A definition of this phase might well be "a placing before the patient of such information as has been gained in this and previous consultations, along with other related information the doctor may feel important, in order to establish some degree of consensual approach to the subsequent stages of the consultation and the future management of the patient's condition".

In nearly 30 per cent of consultations we have on tape it does not occur at all, and in a further 48 per cent it does not occupy one-tenth of the time used in the whole consultation. As will be noted later in the section on styles of consultation, this particular behaviour seems to represent the doctor's beliefs about his patients' ability to involve themselves in their own treatment, and is particularly associated with a non-authoritarian approach to patient management.

It is not quite true to say that this phase either exists in a doctor's consultation or does not exist. It is, however, true to say that some doctors do not even appear to realise its strategic value because they fail to use it even when faced with situations where there would appear to be no other choice. On the basis of the evidence we have it appears that when a doctor uses it consistently it will appear in one shape or another in more than 60 per cent of his consultations. Those doctors with whom it does not appear consistently only appear to use it when dealing with highly articulate patients who demonstrate that they do not view the doctor/patient consultation as a superordinate-subordinate relationship.

Whilst no measure of semantic differential has been applied to patients there is some evidence that those doctors who use the behaviour consistently do not use it with patients who have little command of the language, eg immigrant patients.

An example of this pattern of behaviour would run as follows. The doctor is interviewing a middle-aged man who is an executive in a northern engineering business. The man has been to see a specialist and has returned to his GP for a further examination and to learn the news from the specialist. The examination is complete and the patient has re-entered the consulting room.

D. "Okay, John. Well, I've finished my tests and I've got the report."

P. "Well then, tell me straight out, is it cancer?"

D. "No, it is not cancer, in fact it is nothing of the sort."

P. "Well, thank God for that. You don't know what a load that is off my mind."

D. "Well, it's not cancer and it's not something which is immediately life-

25

threatening. But that's where the good news stops. The tests I've run and Mr Hawker's report are not all that good news. You have a heart condition which will get worse unless we do something. You have a blood-pressure which frankly is not good. You have had an ulcer for years."

P. "It all sounds to me like I'm a middle-aged executive about to become a company liability."

D. "Well, let's look at causes. There are all sorts of theories I could tell you about, but in your case I'm going to give you just a couple which I am certain fit your case. In the first place, you and I have known for two years that you are under more stress than you can take at work. We both know you have not had a holiday these last two years and you have been working all the hours God sends. Right?"

P. "Well, yes. But we've had a bad year or two. It won't be that bad in the future."

D. "Then we have had this running battle with you and your smoking. You tell me you are cutting down, but Doris told me only last week that you are shifting two packs a day. Then there's this eating. You don't now eat all those fats, but you still can't find the time for a lunch. A couple of pints and a butty. Pills to make you sleep. Christ, John, you're in danger of becoming a walking pharmacy. Now what about it."

P. "Well, okay, you're the doc. Spell it out."

D. "No. It's up to you. You know as well as I do what's got to happen. We both know what the facts are. We both know what's got to be done. Now then, let's hear you spell it out for yourself."

This would be regarded as a fairly strong almost confronting approach in which the doctor is very clearly going to place the burden of problem solving on the patient. The next phase in fact was a trading agreement in which the doctor made clear that he was going to prescribe certain treatments as his side of the bargain. The patient, however, was going to spend a lot of time clarifying what he was going to do for his part of the bargain.

There are also much gentler examples of this type of activity. For example, the following interaction took place between a doctor and a female patient, but the real patient was a child who was noisily interrupting the dialogue.

D. "Well, let's see where we are. You say that he won't eat when children ought to eat. But he seems to me to be fairly well fed. In fact he's a little on the heavy side. You say he won't go to sleep unless you or your husband are in the bedroom. He gets up in the middle of the night and comes into your bed and won't rest until he is right in the middle. He refuses to play with other children when you are around and he creates merry hell when you take him to playschool. He is, however, quite a normal child, in fact he is quite bright. Watch out, he's got your handbag. Oh, dear, too late. It's all over the floor."

P. Oh, look what you have done. Now pick it up, come on. Oh, don't throw it over there. Oh, you are a naughty boy. Now put that down. Come on, sit up here whilst I talk to doctor. Well, I don't know what to say about it. All I know is that I'm worried."

D. "Well, if he was ten what would you say to him?"

P. "He would be a right little mummy boy."

D. "Well, what is he now?"

26

P. "Yes, but he's only four. Now stop that, there's a good boy. That's mummy's lipstick. Yes. Give it to me now. Well, do you think I spoil him?"

D. "Well, you said it. You know, many people think that small children are much more cunning than we realise. They sometimes blackmail their parents, and frankly, they can destroy marriages. They do, however, start to place more and more demands on their parents, almost as though they are trying to find out what they can get away with. Well, what do you think of that?"

All through this interview one gets the impression that this very patient doctor wants to throw the child through his consulting-room window. He remained patient to the end, and even after the child knocked his case cards all over the floor.

The most important variable here is vague indeed. What seems to be true is that the doctor has to recognise that many actions he may wish to prescribe may only be executed if the patient actually wishes to execute his instructions. He must also realise that many patients are likely to execute desirable medical decisions if they believe that they have been a party to the making of those decisions.

There is an apocryphal story of a Rochdale doctor who saw an old lady every fortnight for 10 years and regularly prescribed a particular medicine. After her death he visited her house and found 10 years' supply of bottles, all unopened.

V Detailing treatment or further investigation

This phase may well be a long verbal set of instructions to take certain pills and do certain things, or it may be a completely non-verbal, instant tearing-off of a sheet of paper from the prescription pad with the terse message, "Take this to the chemist."

There are not only considerable variations between doctors in the management of this phase but also variations within individual doctors. There is a much greater probability of a long set of instructions at the start of a morning surgery than at the end of that surgery, but evening surgeries seem, on the whole, to operate in reverse. Obviously there are many conditions which require little detailing of instructions, but there are many instances in which doctors do spend the whole of this phase handing out advice and directions which clearly have no practicality in the eyes of the patient. The following is an example of a doctor giving advice to a manual labourer.

D. "Now look here. You're going to have to give up humping those sacks of cement around that site. Can't you find a job driving a van or something?"

P. "But doctor, you don't get jobs like that at my age."

D. "Well, you must realise that all this hard work is doing you no good at all. You must think of doing something lighter. Go off down to the Labour Exchange and see what they can do for you. Or maybe you can find something in a factory. I mean, there must be something you can do which is less taxing than manual labour."

It is sometimes quite astonishing to hear how insensitive some GPs can be to some of their patients. The doctor quoted above confessed quite honestly that he had no idea at all what options were open to a manual labourer, and had never considered the possibility that most men do that sort of work when there is no other choice open to them.

Another area where a few doctors are hopelessly at sea is in their dealings with immigrant patients. There is one recording of a GP, who admittedly had never previously dealt with an immigrant family, soundly berating a father for his lack of dietary knowledge. "You can't just feed a child on rice. Now the child has got to eat eggs, fish, meat, cheese and all sorts of things like that which contain lots of protein. Then there are all sorts of other foods like fruit which are full of good vitamins."

The fact that he might have said something akin to instructing a Jewish family to eat pork had never occurred to him. This sort of problem, however, is probably only a matter of learning. Doctors who have large immigrant numbers on their lists tend to become expert in their dealings with immigrants and even more careful in their prescribing behaviour than they might be with British patients.

One statistic which is significant in this context concerns the incidence of a patient's "By the way, doctor". This takes many forms but the message is still the same. It might be something like "While I'm here, doctor" or "My sister asked me . . .", but often it turns out to be the real reason for their being there in the first place. The first 1,000 consultations were checked for this sort of occurrence and it was found that there were 79 clear cases over which there could be no doubt. Of these 79, 56 occurred during Phase V. It is in all senses a parting shot and a cause of considerable doctor frustration. As we shall observe in the chapter on dysfunction, it clearly has some relationship to Phase II.

VI Terminating

This is simply the way in which the doctor indicates that it is time for the patient to go. By far the most potent indicator of termination is the tearing-off of the prescription. This produces almost a conditioned response in the patient. Other doctors have direct word forms like "Off you go now" or "Off you go to the chemist and get this filled out". Some doctors actually stand up and walk to the door whilst a few call in the next patient and then say goodbye. Like relating to the patient this pattern of doctor behaviour is remarkably consistent with the majority of his patients and only rarely does it change.

In about 10 per cent of all consultations we have studied the patient appears to initiate the termination, but there is usually some sort of signal like the handing over of a piece of paper which seems to start the process. This is, in fact, the only part of the consultation, with the exception of very rare instances of patients relating to the doctor before he gets a chance, in which the patient actually does play a significant role in initiation. In the overwhelming majority of all other phases the initiation of a new phase is performed by the doctor.

We have had discussions as to whether or not the "by the way" is a genuine example of patient initiation. It certainly indicates that what the doctor is doing is not what the patient wishes him to do, while it is certainly an opportunity for the patient to take over the control of the consultation. Doctors seem to have a limited number of strategies for coping with this sort of event:

(a) Ignore it.

(b) Defer or temporise.

(c) Cope.

Coping also comes in two forms:

(i) Complete reversion to Phase II.

(ii) Short-term management within the context of Phases V or VI.

28

There is no clear-cut picture of how doctors react to such a situation. A few take a very hard line and refuse to deal with such interventions under any circumstances. They claim that the patient is not playing the game according to the rules and must therefore suffer the penalty. Most appear to prefer options (b) or (c)(ii) but occasionally will take the (c)(i) option. This latter course of action is more likely to happen in an evening surgery than a morning surgery.

All this describes a sequence of events which may be observed in the doctor/patient consultation. What must be added is that this sequence does not occur in all consultations, only in 63 per cent. It is also true that only some parts of this sequence occur in most consultations and with some doctors some parts never occur at all. A large number of consultations are, of course, only incomplete acts in a very long drama. Repeat prescriptions, for example, include Phases I, V and VI because on the whole Phases II, III and possibly IV have taken place on a previous occasion. Equally, would-be tourists requiring various injections/inoculations usually go through Phases I, II, V and VI.

There is also a further problem that this ideal sequence does not always follow its own progression. There are many consultations in which the interview progresses as far as Phase V only to have to return to Phase II. There is even one extensive consultation in which the sequence runs I, II, V, II, III, V, II, V, II, III, V, VI, II, VI.

In most circumstances it would be normal to find that five of the phases are to be found in all long new cases (see Taylor), the omission being Phase IV. This set of events also seems to occur irrespective of most of the factors which might influence a consultation. For example, it occurs in all geographical settings and as far as can be seen is independent of the variable of illness. The only real constraint, apart from the probable absence of Phase IV, is the issue of language. With immigrant patients working through an interpreter, Phase II is often run into Phase III as soon as the doctor gets some sort of lead.

What is useful about this analysis is that most of the questions, answers and statements made in a consultation can be related to where the doctor appears to be in this sequence. As the doctor controls the evolution of this sequence of events (often apparently unconsciously) he may be observed to be attempting to follow some sort of routine. If he has progressed through his examination of the patient and is detailing treatment and then suddenly asks a diagnostic question or even a question about why the patient is there at all, he is moving the consultation back in sequence because he is not satisfied with the position he has.

The analysis also gives us a process check on the development of the strategy of a consultation, and allows all consultations to be analysed against this yardstick. We may then, for example, observe that a particular doctor never uses Phase IV or that doctors using extensive amounts of time in Phase II appear to get through Phases III, V and VI very quickly.

There is also the fact that most of the events which take place in a consultation are governed by the doctor's perception of where he thinks he is in the development of a consultation. In 95 per cent of all consultations studied it may be safely argued that the doctor is in charge of the "how" of that consultation as well as the "what". Even when the doctor opts to use a non-directive patient-oriented strategy it is the doctor who makes that decision and not the patient.

CHAPTER 4
THE MINUTIAE OF THE CONSULTATION
THE OVERTURE
PART I

Having identified that consultations appear to have some sort of structure or sequence of events, the research moved on to an analysis of the degree to which the verbal behaviour of the doctor could also be categorised. In this particular area there are several useful guidelines in a number of disciplines. Some of these have already been noted in Chapter 1.

The best-known analysis of interactive behaviour is probably that of R F Bales.[7] He has devised a 12-factor system of examining group behaviour which suggests that in group situations most of the behaviours may be grouped under the following headings:

(a) Asking for information
(b) Giving information
(c) Asking for opinion
(d) Giving opinion
(e) Asking for suggestions
(f) Making suggestions
(g) Agreeing
(h) Disagreeing
(i) Increasing tension
(j) Decreasing tension
(k) Integration
(l) Disintegration.

Items (a) to (f) are described as "task-oriented behaviours" and items (g) to (l) are described as "process-oriented behaviours".

Bales' system was successful in so far as it identified a manageable number of measurements. Some previous research had involved 300 or more items of behaviour, which made any serious observation almost impossible. The weakness of Bales' approach, however, is that it does not have enough sensitivity. Early attempts in this research to apply this approach to the doctor/patient consultations proved inadequate, if only because much doctor behaviour falls under the broad heading of "questioning", ie items (a) and (c). It allows little room, for example, to distinguish between "open-ended questions" and "closed questions". In the research the ability to be able to make such distinctions is of particular importance.

There are also a number of ways of categorising teacher behaviour which are used extensively, especially the work of Flanders.[14] None of these systems, however, really solves the problem of the doctor/patient consultation because they are all based upon the workings of groups of more than five or six people. Most doctor/patient interactions are made up of not more than two people, and very rarely are there more than three people in the consulting-room. The same problem applies to the more recent developments in this field such as Rackham and Honey's[15] approach to developing interactive skills.

The basic problem thus presented by the doctor/patient relationship was that no extant pattern of interaction could be used as a basis and there were few research insights into the nature of interaction in the diadic situation. Clearly then, it was necessary to attempt some classification of doctor behaviour, but this classification has to fulfil certain requirements:

(a) It should contain sufficient variety of categories to allow for a reasonable degree of behavioural delineation.

(b) It should be capable of being used by a single observer working preferably from cheap available systems of recording, ie audio-tape casette recorders.

(c) It should be capable of development into a teaching instrument, which can be used by trained GP teachers as a developmenta Instrument for their trainees and for themselves.

The definition of what constitutes a "behaviour" is quite complex. Some researchers prefer to split all communication into five- or three-second units and to place a definition upon that activity which takes place within that period of time. Whilst this is a very useful research technique it is not really helpful to the would-be teacher because of the complexity of analysis involved in this method.

The method used here is the same as the method used by Hays and Larson[8] in their study of nurses, namely "units of sense". Take the following excerpt from a consultation: "Now then, Mrs X, first of all, these pains occurred when you were walking for long periods and then they started to occur when you were doing your normal housework and now they are occurring even when you climb stairs. Is that right?"

This interaction actually lasted for more than 10 seconds. Thus a five-second approach would split it into two parts and label Part 1 a statement and Part 2 a question. A three-second approach would list two statements and then a question. In fact, however, the sense of this collection of words is quite unitary. The doctor is recapitulating a set of data given by the patient and is attempting to put that data into a correct sequence. The question at the end is simply to check whether or not the data is correctly sequenced. If the reply is "Yes" then the doctor has achieved the correct sequence. If the reply is "No", then he has to find some way of getting the sequence right.

A further assumption made in this research is that the doctor/patient consultation is a goal-seeking activity in which, while each party has goals, the goals of one party may or may not be clear to the other party. The doctor will assume that something has caused the patient to come to his surgery. His assumption may be based upon some previous meeting and thus he will spend little or no time confirming his assumption. His assumption may be based upon his views of the practice of medicine, thus he will seek to make the patient fit into a format he wishes to impose upon patients. Alternatively he will investigate the patient's apparent reasons for being there and allow the goals of the consultation to be determined largely by the patient.

Utilising these assumptions and the "unit of sense" model described previously, we may then proceed to view the consultation as a simple pattern of activity, namely, objective-strategy-tactics. Each unit of sense thus becomes a tactic and collections of tactics give us insights into the doctor's sense of strategy.

Using this model to analyse consultations a number of observations may be made which are dealt with variously later in this work.

(a) There appear to be a large number of consultations in which the content may be described as "organic" in which the doctors appear to achieve a diagnosis comparatively easily. The verbal behaviours used are fairly straightforward, using direct and closed questions, correlational questions and often some physical examinations. A good example of this appears to be the routine ante-natal examination.

(b) There appear to be a smaller number of consultations in which the content is not wholly organic and confusion is observed when the doctor attempts to define the purpose of the activity using the tactics he has developed in his approach to organic situations.

(Confusion was observed on a number of occasions when the doctor and the patient appear not to be talking about the same thing, or when both appear to be talking at the same time or in which there is no apparent sequence between question and answer.)

(c) We found a limited number of consultations in which the doctor and the patient appeared to achieve total dysfunction, and all such consultations dealt with family problems. The patient and the doctor indulge in quite odd behaviour. The patient replies to direct questions with statements about some other issue which is not shared with the doctor. The doctor persists with the same approach and a situation develops in which the doctor pursues a strategy regardless of the patient and the patient pursues a consultation regardless of the doctor. Apart from their physical presence together in a room there is no other point of contact between the parties.

In order to investigate the consultation, further various ways were tried of analysing what takes place. The most fruitful initial approach came from an analysis of behaviours which occurred consistently during phases of the consultation (see Chapter 3).

This produced a list of behaviours which was capable of describing at least 60 per cent of all the interaction in a consultation, but it did not altogether allow the analysis of behaviour in a developmental fashion because some behaviours recur frequently in other parts of the consultation.

However, one area which provided useful insights was a short study of the events which take place as soon as a patient enters the doctor's consulting-room. One of the most interesting features of this study was the consistent way in which doctors manage this situation. Some, for example, repeat the same words on almost 90 per cent of all occasions. Typical of this standardised opening is the following: "Good morning Mr/Mrs/Miss —— and what can we do for you today?" Or one GP in London who uses the following word form for at least 70 per cent of his patients: "Hullo, Mrs —— and what can we do you for?"

Some GPs vary their opening remarks according to the sex of the patient and appear to adopt much more friendly tones when greeting female patients, and one GP in fact completely changed his accent when talking to female patients.

It was possible to classify most of the behaviours used in relating to patients. Basically these fall under the following headings:

(1) Giving recognition

For example, "Good morning, Mrs Smith, and how are you today?" or "Hello, Mrs Black, you do look well." This behaviour is observed when a patient is already known to the doctor. To be able to give recognition depends upon either the doctor's good memory or the effectiveness of his medical records.

When the doctor does not know the patient, but has a clear indication of who it might be, ie from an appointment register or from a record card, giving recognition assumes a rather different form: for example, "Good morning (pause), you are Mrs Smith, aren't you?" This type of behaviour will be referred to below. (See (4).)

(2) Offering self

This form of relating to patients differs from the above simply because the doctor, instead of offering recognition of the patient, offers himself. For example, "Hello, please sit down. I am Dr Jones" or "Hello, and what can I do for you today?"

NB. Some consultations take place between three persons. The most common three-person consultation involves a mother and child (57 per cent of sample trios are mother and child). Less frequently husband and wife (11 per cent almost invariably pensioners) and less frequently still immigrants with interpreters (4 per cent). With a mother/child trio it appears to be very common practice to relate to the child first and then the mother. For example, "Hello, Jimmy. My, my, you are growing into a big boy. And what is it that brings you both here today, Mrs X?"

These two patterns describe most of the openings doctors use when meeting patients (70 per cent). There are, however, some doctors who use much less personal forms of opening. It also appears that doctors who are, on the whole, "self offerers" use a similar form of opening with some patients. Where it has been possible to follow up these doctors it has been noted that on the whole they change their style of opening when they dislike the patient sitting in front of them. These openings are described here as:

(3) Impersonal openings

Occasionally consultations in which the doctor and the patient do not appear to bother with any of the normal rituals of social behaviour. For example, "Come in. Sit down. Now then, what is it today?" This approach is, as will be noted, an immediate entry to what has been suggested as Phase II of a consultation (see Chapter 3).

Another doctor suggested that he might use such an approach when he felt that he was falling behind his schedule. He felt, despite the absence of any evidence, that it was a much shorter way of getting to the point.

It has already been noted above that there is a variation on the theme of "giving recognition". This could well be listed as:

(4) Seeking recognition

In the pilot sample there were two doctors who were fairly new to their practice, and therefore had few established relationships to work with. Commonly they used a form of relating similar to the following: "Good morning. Now, you are Mr Smith, is that right?" It has also been noted that both these doctors subsequently have changed their approach as they have developed relationships.

(5) Apologising

This is a not uncommon way of opening a consultation when the doctor is

33

behind his schedule. "Good morning. I am sorry to have kept you waiting. Now what can I do for you?"

Occasionally this behaviour will be noted when doctors realise that they have made mistakes. "I am sorry. I have been looking at the wrong notes."

Occasionally the information given to a doctor before the patient arrives is the wrong information. Frequently this will not become apparent until the consultation has advanced very considerably. In one case, involving immigrant patients, the doctor discovered that he was conducting a physical examination of the wrong patient. However, it can occur at the very start of an interview. This would lead to the definition of a category of:

(6) Dysfunctional openings

There were several instances of dysfunctional openings, the most common being a consequence of bad information supply from a receptionist. Twenty-three instances of the following type of opening were noted: "You don't look like Mr Smith, Miss umm umm; I think I have the wrong cards."

Equally, in areas where there are a few common surnames a doctor will make a mistake and completely ruin his opening gambit. For example:
D. "Hullo, Mrs McCullough. How's the little boy?"
P. "What little boy?"

Another form of apparent dysfunction occurs quite frequently when doctors continue to write patient notes for the previous patient when a new patient has arrived. "Sit down, please. I am just finishing writing these cards. I won't be a minute or two." Or, "Just sit over there, would you? I must fill in these bits of card."

This is dysfunctional in the sense that it has nothing to do with the problem of the new patient, although it may have something to do with the problems of the doctor. Some patients seem quite unmoved by the experience whilst others who are perhaps more anxious do make some attempts to say things when the doctor is writing. It can also lead to situations like the following:
D. "Good morning. The weather is nice outside, isn't it? Sit down, I'm just finishing these notes."
P. "It is raining."
D. "That's nice."

Discussion with this particular doctor revealed that he was busy writing notes when the patient was sent in from the waiting-room. Instead of the usual gap of about 20 seconds the patient must have sprinted and thus not allowed the doctor to complete his record-keeping routines. He had no recall of the actual interaction.

Little is to be gained by any further study of the way in which doctors greet their patients. On the whole it would appear to be a completely idiosyncratic matter and apart from its predictability it offers little to the researcher or would-be teacher.

What happens next, however, is very significant. As we shall observe in a later section, discovering the real reason for the patient being there is a vital activity.

As may be observed, most forms of relating to a patient have the effect of inviting the patient to give the doctor the basic information he needs in order to progress. There are, however, many other ways of advancing the consultation, ranging from telling the patient why he is there to making some oblique reference to a possible reason for attendance.

(7) Telling—a comparatively rare behaviour. (Giving information)

"Now, you've come for that prescription" or "You want some more of that medicine again. Right?"

Almost inevitably this type of statement relates to previous experience or to some aspect of the on-going relationship between a GP and his patient. No case was discovered on our tapes of a GP actually telling a stranger why he or she was there, although two doctors have separately reported the story of a doctor who was capable of this. Apparently this particular GP could "smell the disease" as it came through the door. Olfactory approaches to patients unfortunately do not appear on tape recordings.

(8) Relating to some previous experience

A more common form of working through an on-going consultation is as follows:

For example:

"Now, you were in last week."

"We decided last month that you ought to come back today, didn't we?"

The effect of this behaviour seems to be to encourage the patient to tell the doctor whether or not the cause of the previous meeting was the same as the cause of this meeting. Discussion with practitioners suggests that this question is valuable because it allows the doctor to avoid repetition if the reason for both consultations is the same.

Alternatively, if it is not the same reason he knows that he has to deal with more than one issue. Equally, it may also suggest to the doctor the probability of a missed diagnosis and the need for re-examination.

Three other approaches to opening up the consultation have been observed. Whilst the form of words may not be quite the same, in nearly all cases the generic descriptions offered cover most of the options open to a doctor not using the above.

(9) Direct questions

For example:

"What is wrong with you today?"

"What's hurting today, and where is it?"

This approach seeks to focus the patient's attention directly on a specific reason for attendance. It is very much a feature of those doctors who achieve a short consultation time. The latter example is apparently only used by doctors who are working within an established relationship, and who, by their tone of voice, indicate whether the patient and the doctor enjoy a good-humoured relationship, or whether the doctor is seeking to express some impatience.

(10) Broad opening

For example:

"Is there something you would like to talk to me about?"

"Where would you like to begin?"

"What can I do for you today?"

35

This approach is very typical of GPs with a low consultation rate. The reaction to the broad opening, however, indicates that some doctors with a short consultation time may also use the broad opening. When coupled with behaviour "encouraging" (see below) it is very probable that the consultation could last a long time.

(11) Offering observation

For example:
"You appear to be very tense today."
"You are not sitting very comfortably."
"You have been crying."
"My goodness me, you are upset."

This behaviour has a similar effect to the direct question, but apparently no question has been asked. It is also used most frequently by those doctors who achieve a low consultation rate. Its effect is to focus the attention of the patient upon the causes which might underly tension or tears. Coupled with "silence" (see below) it also precedes a lot of patient participation and little doctor participation.

In this context it is worth noting two other aspects of behaviour which may appear very early in a consultation, especially if the doctor has opted to use the last two behaviours (broad opening and offering observation). These behaviours are described as:

(12) Encouraging

For example:
"Go on."
"Tell me more."
"Uh, uh."

The examples given are only a few of the various noises doctors use to encourage patients to keep talking. Some doctors sound as though they are grunting whilst others "Mmmmmmmm" endlessly.

(13) Using silence

Very few of the interactionists have really studied the use of silence, although Sanhammer et al[16] note that it occupies an important part of the therapeutic side of the nurse/patient relationship.[7] Various studies of interviewing technique have also concluded that silence can be a most valuable tool in the hands of a competent interviewer.[16]

Within the doctor/patient relationship the use of silence is infrequent except with a small percentage of doctors (7 per cent) who use it consistently. During the validation of parts of this research several groups of doctors considered the issue of silence and offered reasons for not using it. These may be listed in order of frequency as below:

(a) Time pressure is too great in a five- or six-minute schedule.
(b) The tension upon the patient is too great.
(c) If the doctor remains silent the patient will remain silent.
(d) The tension on the doctor is too great.

There is a strong correlation between those doctors who do use silence regularly and those doctors who have been influenced by the late Michael

Balint. They accept Balint's premise that patients are obliged to play a certain game in order to enter the surgery, and the doctors are thus prepared to spend time cutting through the smokescreen in order to discover the real reasons behind a patient's attendance.[9]

Some of the doctors using the "broad opening" as a technique to get the patient to verbalise the real reason for attendance demonstrate a need to keep the patient talking until such clues as the patient cares to offer are detected by the doctor. Discussion with exponents of this behaviour reveals a strongly held belief that patients confronted with direct questions at the start of a consultation rarely give complete answers. By forcing the patient to talk, it is claimed that the process of relationship building is continued to the point where the patient feels sufficiently confident to make the real purpose of the visit apparent.

Consequently one may examine "encouragement" and "silence" as two possible strategies which may open up the patient. All of this is naturally based to a large extent upon beliefs about the nature of medicine and beliefs about patients. To advocate a Balint type model raises many medical hackles. There is a school of thought which considers the GP to be a keeper of physiological health and nothing else. Another view is that the doctor must firstly ensure that the patient has no organic illness before delving into any more remote area of the patient's life. To some extent it is possible to indicate the beliefs of a particular doctor simply by observing his behaviour.

This short section is simply a review of what might happen during the first minute or so of a consultation. The route taken is important because so much of what follows appears to be determined by the first few seconds. A greeting followed by a few short direct questions will probably lead very quickly into a diagnostic and prescribing mode of behaviour and hence to a quick and early termination of the consultation. A greeting followed by an observation, however, will produce a totally different avenue and a longer consultation.

During one part of the research it was possible to examine three patients, attending the same practice but meeting different doctors. One of the patients met two doctors who worked at almost extreme poles of the patient/doctor centred spectrum. In one case the interview lasted for four minutes whilst in the other case it lasted for nine minutes. The diagnosis of the condition and the treatment prescribed were totally different. What is more important is the fact that what the patient said to one doctor was not the same as was said to the other—yet the presented symptoms were identical.

CHAPTER 5
THE MINUTIAE OF THE CONSULTATION
PART II

In the previous chapter we concentrated upon the opening few seconds of a consultation in which the doctor was attempting to relate to the patient and to explore the question of why the patient was there. As we have observed, the greeting itself is quite idiosyncratic but what follows is very much related to the style of the doctor (see Chapters 9 and 10).

As was noted earlier, consultations develop from this point in a variety of ways. Here we are concerned with those things a doctor may say which will lead him from the point at which he believes he knows why the patient is there to the point where he is about to prescribe some future course of action. This section is, in fact, largely concerned with the activity of examining patients, and making some sort of diagnosis.

When a patient has enunciated some description of symptoms, the doctor is then faced with the task of advancing this pattern of knowledge from whatever crude form it happens to take into a set of data which will allow him to make some intelligent guess at the condition.

One of the great problems of this research was attempting to study the sorts of things patients may say to doctors. The task, in fact, proved to be too great, although a brief attempt at semantic differential tests suggested that such a line of research might prove useful. Sadly we were not in a position to apply such tests to the patients we studied.

During an influenza epidemic many patients came and went with almost identical symptoms, yet the presentation of these symptoms was quite different. For example:

D. "Good morning, Mr Y. You seem to be running away with something or other."

P. "Well, I've got a bad cold, a temperature of 101, a foul headache and a lot of vague aches in my leg muscles. I assume that I have influenza and have come here for you to confirm that fact."

D. "Well, there is a lot about at the moment. . . ."

P. "And I look like another, right?"

D. "Well, yes, you do in fact. . . ."

P. "And there's nothing you can really do, is there?"

D. "Well, I can tell you to go to bed and take it easy and I can give you something to ease the symptoms. The body itself, however, will take care of the influenza in its own good time. I suppose I can give you the statistical odds on it killing you, if you want."

P. "Well, that's fine. I'll go off to bed for three or four days. I'll take your panegyrics, and if I fail to die but also fail to recover in three days I'll be in touch."

D. "Well, here's your bit of paper. If I were you I would buy a bottle of rum. It won't do you any good but you'll feel better. Cheerio."

Compare that patient with the following example, in which the next patient on that particular GP's appointment list behaved as follows:

D. "Good morning, Mrs J——. My goodness me, you've got a shocker."

P. "Oh, I'm not well doctor."

D. "Well, I can see you have a cold. Anything else?"

P. "Well, I'm not good at all. I've got a pain here."

D. "A headache?"

P. "Well, not like I normally have, you know. I mean, this one is all over my eyes and down the side here. I've got a right one here. I said to my husband this morning. . . ."

D. "Do you have any aches?"

P. "Well, you know me. I've got pains all the time."

D. "Yes, but do you have any new pains?"

P. "Eh? Well, aye. Down here."
D. "Do you have a temperature?"
P. "Well, I must have. I mean, I'm sweating something terrible."
D. "Have you actually taken your temperature?"
P. "No. I've nothing."
D. "Right. Well now, pop this into your mouth, will you? Mmmmm."
P. "What is it then?"
D. "Yes, you have a temperature."

Consultation No 1 was complete within two minutes, whilst consultation No 2 took six-and-a-half minutes. The first example is also interesting because it is one of the few doctor/patient consultations in which the bulk of the initiative comes from the patient. The problem with attempting to categorise the things patients say is made confusing by virtue of the fact that verbal ranges are so different, as is an understanding of sickness.

The doctor, on the other hand, is much more consistent. In the above example, although the doctor used slightly different word forms, in fact he used the same pattern of behaviour of opening up a consultation with a clear observation of what the trouble might be.

When the doctor has some idea of what the patient thinks has brought him to the surgery, the doctor will then begin to display his interrogative technique. The way in which questions are asked by doctors is remarkably consistent. Below is a list of a range of question types noted in the research, with examples.

(14) Closed questions
For example:

"Do you have a pain here?"
"Do you have a headache?"

These are similar questions to direct questions (see above) but are characterised by complete specificity and a preference for yes or no answers.

(15) Open-ended questions (see "Broad opening" above)
A similar observation may be made here. This sort of question is almost invariably associated with a low consultation rate. In general, however, it is not quite as non-specific as the broad opening, because it occurs at a stage when the development of the consultation is becoming clear. The following two examples indicate how a combination of specificity by the doctor, whilst allowing free range to the patient, can be seen to work.

For example:

"Would you like to talk about this stress at work?"
"Tell me about these pains, will you?"

In both of these examples it is clear that the doctor is pursuing some information already gleaned. However, he is allowing the patient to select what is important within the area offered.

One observation which might be made at this point concerns the adage, "The shorter the question the longer the answer and vice versa." This adage is misleading. Short direct questions produce short answers. Short open-ended questions produce long answers.

39

(16) Placing events in some time, place or sequence

For example:

"What seemed to lead up to this?"

"Was it before or after?"

"When did that happen?"

"Has it happened before?"

These appear to be a very important part of making a diagnosis, and tend to be used as supplementary questions.

(17) Correlational questions

For example:

"Does this pain come on after you have been running?"

"Do you suffer from this pain after you have been drinking?"

These questions are similar to those in (16) above, but seek to relate a symptom to a specific activity rather than to a time or place.

(18) Rhetorical questions

For example:

"That was a silly thing to do, wasn't it?"

These are basically not questions at all but some sort of value judgement which the doctor wishes to make. They are usually associated with critical behaviour. This sort of question also appears to be a useful short cut with some patients.

For example:

"Now you have got a pain here haven't you? Of course you have."

In print some of the natural "loading" is lost and the reader will have to experiment in order to get the values right.

In many ways the rhetorical question causes a problem, because it is so often used as an instrument to chastise patients (see below). In making a judgement on which type of behaviour it might be, one is forced to rely upon the context of the behaviour and the past performance of the doctor. The rhetorical question is also used by some doctors as a "shut out". Often a patient will volunteer some information when the doctor does not want the information and he will use the rhetorical question to stop the patient.

For example, in the following extract a female patient, 50, is on the point of being referred to a specialist. The doctor has made this line of action clear much earlier in the consultation. He is then patiently going over all of his information.

D. "Now then, you will go up to see Mr Chisholm at the hospital and you will take this note with you. I will write to him to confirm the appointment. Now then, you must tell him all that you have told me, even if he appears to ask you questions which I have asked. In particular try to remember all that you told me about your waking up after the attack."

P. "Did I tell you our John had an accident last week?"

D. "Well, that was careless of him, wasn't it? Now then, back to Mr Chisholm."

(19) Hidden questions

For example:

"That holiday must have done you a lot of good. We must talk about it some time."

40

"Well, I expect that if you do decide to change your job things might improve at home."

These questions sound like statements which demand no immediate response. But the response which they often do produce is the same as the answer to an open-ended question. When it is possible to identify such questions, they should be so recorded. Difficulty has been experienced in identifying this behaviour. In the last resort it depends upon the response of the patient. If, in the first example above, the patient were to reply "Yes" and no more, then its classification would be problematic.

(20) Reflected questions

For example:

P. "Do you think I am silly to feel like that?"
D. "Do you think you are silly?"
or
P. "Do you think I should change my job?"
D. "How do you feel about changing your job?"

The reflected question is an easily identifiable and specific skill. Curiously it is one of those behaviours which is either present in quantity or not present at all. It does not seem to exist in half measures. It is also possible to observe that it exists as part of a composite package in company with such behaviours as "clarifying", "seeking patient ideas", "using patient ideas". (See below.)

These categories cover most of the types of questioning a doctor may use. Questions, however, are not the only part of his diagnostic armoury. Question forms, however, do give us a lot of insight into the way in which a doctor sees his patients. Some doctors use a near standard battery of short questions and require short answers. These doctors, on the whole, as we will observe later, can terminate a consultation very quickly and symbolically by tearing off a piece of paper and offering no explanation, only a set of instructions.

Those doctors using the reflected question show two quite dissimilar tendencies. Some, about 40 per cent of those using the behaviour, will continue to follow a modified counselling model right through to the end of the consultation. Others, and this represents the majority, appear to use the reflected question as a device to enable them to achieve a much more accurate diagnosis. They will not, however, use much patient-centred behaviour once they have made a diagnosis.

In addition to questioning skills the following behaviours have been observed to be particularly common during the process leading up to a diagnosis.

(21) Exploring

For example:

"Tell me more about that."
"Will you describe that in more detail?"

These behaviours are similar in some ways to (22) (below), and indeed in any simple teaching model they could well be placed under the same heading. There is, however, one procedure in which exploration and suggestion (see below) combine in an interesting fashion.

For example:

P. "Nobody understands me."

41

D. "Do you mean you cannot talk to me?"
or
P. "Nobody takes any notice of me."
D. "You mean your wife ignores you?"

(22) Clarifying

For example:
"I am not sure that I understand what you are saying to me. Please try again."

This is a behaviour which may frequently occur when dealing with immigrant patients or indeed native population who suffer from an inability to verbalise clearly.

(23) Suggesting

For example:
P. "When I lie down I feel all funny."
D. "You mean you go dizzy?"
P. "When I am running about the house doing all the housework, I get all flustered and short-tempered. . . ."
D. "You mean you get out of breath quickly?"

NB. (22) and (23) are very difficult to distinguish from each other in some instances. What has been observed, however, is the frequency with which "suggesting" is used in an effort to move the consultation into a post-diagnostic phase. It seems likely that suggestion may well be a short-cut route which enables the doctor to develop the consultation more quickly. This, however, is not a general rule.

When used with (20) and (21) it can be seen as a supportive device which enables patients who have difficulty in verbalising problems to sustain a difficult and introspective self-analysis.

(24) Indicating understanding

For example:
"I see."
or
"I follow."
or
"Uh-hu."

These behaviours are very similar to those recorded under "encouraging". What has been observed, however, is a subtle difference in purpose. Doctors using "encouraging" also use "reflecting" when they are trying to get a patient to focus upon a specific issue. Doctors who use the behaviour labelled "indicating understanding" simply follow the flow of what a patient is saying and do not in any way attempt to direct or control. When the patient has finished the doctor then simply carries on in control of the situation, whereas the "encourager" is quite prepared to allow the patient to decide upon the speed with which the consultation flows.

(25) Miscellaneous professional noises

There still existed, on tape, a collection of noises rather than words which

42

appeared to have no real meaning. Whilst a patient may be encouraged with a grunt or some other noise, and equally a doctor may indicate understanding with some sort of noise or other, there are still noises which could not be categorised in either of these two areas. In most cases it was possible to observe that these noises were made when a doctor was actually undertaking a physical examination of the patient, and in particular when he was examining the patient's back. On questioning it was discovered that most doctors are quite unaware of these curious noises, but later they reported that the noises were related to bits of a physical examination. For example, whilst listening to parts of the lung a doctor would grunt when he had finished the top of the lung and was moving on to a lower point. In all cases the doctors questioned were able to state that the noises were in no way of importance to them and were not intended for patient consumption. Consequently these were listed as "misc. prof. noises".

One curious habit was observed under this heading. One doctor, whilst listening to a patient's chest, would suddenly start to make noises, bom-boom, bom-boom, bom-boom. This was done apparently in rhythm with the patient's heart beat. In this case the doctor concerned was aware of this habit and ascribed it to a period in his life when he was partially deaf. He would pick up the heart beat rhythm "in the good ear and then just in case it got lost would keep it up". He claimed that he had become so accurate in this habit that he could detect various abnormalities in this fashion.

A final behaviour found in the diagnostic stage is:

(26) Doubting

For example:

"Don't you think that's a little strange?"

"Really?"

"I find that very hard to believe."

Doubting is a very odd behaviour in so far as it is used frequently but seems to attract exactly the opposite result to the expected. It seems to be used when the doctor considers that the patient is over-exaggerating or even fantasising. The result, however, in about 60 per cent of instances was to encourage the patient to defend what had been said, rather than to qualify it. Also, one should note in this context two further behaviours which do not lend themselves to any sort of example:

(27) Listening

(28) Using silence

It is very obvious in some tapes that doctors occasionally do not listen to the total amount of information given by a patient. Quite frequently one hears patients being asked for information they have already given, and even more often one hears the same question being put twice. Interrupting a patient is also another symptom of the selective listening doctor. Given the pressures of a busy surgery it is quite possible to understand why doctors wish to hurry patients, but one is bound to suspect that the little pieces of information which are shut out may have some validity.

With these behaviour patterns doctors usually progress an interview to the point where they are capable of making some diagnosis. There is no order in which the questions may be asked and no set sequence. There are, however, patterns.

Closed questions often recur in company with correlational questions and suggestions.

Open-ended questions tend to be associated with placing events in time, place, or sequence and exploring.

As we shall observe later on, there is quite a clear-cut pattern of style observable in GP behaviour, and the recurrence of distinct patterns of interviewing is only a reflection of a consistency of style.

So far we have concentrated on the behaviours which are typical of those patterns prior to the doctor actually coming to some sort of conclusion about the condition of the patient. There is a point in the consultation when the doctor mentally makes some sort of decision. That decision might be a clear diagnosis, it might be an inspired guess, or it may well be a recognition that he is not going to make any sort of diagnosis at all. Equally the decision might be to refer the problem to one of the various specialist services offered. We now focus upon what happens after that point.

When a doctor is conducting a physical examination he will indicate that he has finished by the ritual washing of hands, and if he has made some sort of decision there will be some other near ritual he goes through prior to actually saying anything to the patient. Some GPs clear their throat as they walk back to their desks, whilst others shuffle pieces of paper upon their desks.

There are also many verbal conjunctions used to tie the consultation together. These are usually idiosyncratic but none the less very consistent. For example, many doctors use the expression "now then . . ." to complete one part of the consultation and progress to another. An attempt was made to categorise these conjunctions but was not pursued, due again to the idiosyncrasy of the subject.

We have not really considered what doctors may do when the initiative has been taken by patients. Whilst this is a comparatively rare phenomenon there do exist a group of patients who initiate and sustain the initiative in consultations. The following is an example of one type of initiative taking:

D. "Come in."
P. "Oh, hello doctor. Oh, I am rotten. . . ."
D. "Well, now. . . ."
P. "How I got here, I don't know. . . ."
D. ". . . what can I. . . ."
P. "I feel right rotten."
D. (Obviously giving up an unequal battle) "So do I, now then. . . ."
P. "It started this morning . . ." etc.

Normally this particular doctor has time to manage the following opening:
   "Well now, Mrs X, and what can I do for you today?" when he knew the patient.

When he did not know the patient he used the following:
   "Good morning Mr Y. It is Mr Y, isn't it? I'm Dr J——. And what can I do for you today?"

In this example the doctor resigned himself to losing the initiative and made little attempt to get it back until he had been given a long and lurid account of the development of a cold.

Other doctors are quite unwilling to allow patients to take any initiative at all.

44

The following is the content of a consultation provided by one of the GPs attending a micro-training course at Manchester. He felt quite proud of his control of the patient:

D. "Good morning. I'm Dr G——. Please sit down."

P. "Well, now, I'm only a visitor to this part but I've got something wrong with me, so I thought I ought to come down and get a prescription. All I need is some metarium(?)."

D. "I do not issue prescriptions like that. I will examine you, listen to your symptoms and then will prescribe what I think you need."

P. "I have been taking these now for a few years."

D. "Yes, I'm sure. Now then, please tell me what are your symptoms?"

It might be useful at this stage to examine some of the behaviours doctors use when the initiative has moved to the patient.

(29) Answering patient questions

For example:

P. "Do these spots come up because of the pills?"

D. "I am not sure, but it is possible."

or

D. "That's very likely."

Patients start asking about a diagnosis often before the doctor has made it. This sort of question may well occur at an early stage in the consultation. In this respect what has been observed is a patient asking for a consideration of his condition. Occasionally patients have been observed entering the consultation and simply confronting the doctor with a demand for a diagnosis before anything else has taken place.

For example:

D. "Come in, sit down. Now you are Mrs X."

P. "Yes, have I got 'flu doctor?"

D. "Is that why you have come to see me?"

P. "Well, have I got 'flu or haven't I?"

(30) Evading patient questions

For example:

P. "Have I got TB, doctor?"

D. "I would like you to have an X-ray."

Evasion is a common behaviour observed to a degree in the behaviour of all the doctors in the sample. Sometimes it occurs in a disguised form.

For example:

P. "Have I got something seriously wrong, doctor?"

D. "Well, do you think you have something wrong?"

It seems to be used when the doctor has difficulty in explaining the condition or when he does not want to commit himself or even when he feels he does not want to share his insights with the patient. The first example above is a fairly effective form of evasion because the answer does seem to relate to the question even though it does not answer the question. Rarely does it occur in a much cruder form as below:

P. "Does this mean I will have to give up work?"

D. "What tablets did I prescribe last time?"

(31) Accepting patient ideas

For example:
"That's an interesting idea, we might like to look at it"
or
"Yes, I think that would do you good."

(32) Using patient ideas

For example:
"If that's what you think you would like to do, how do you think you might manage?"

NB. (31) and (32) are clearly identified with those doctors who try to apply the idea that patients may well be able to solve problems for themselves, rather than expecting the doctor to provide solutions for them. As the literature in this field is fairly well developed, the ideas are quite familiar to the medical profession. What is more interesting, however, is the finding that these behaviours are either practised frequently or not used at all. There are several instances of patients offering ideas to doctors who consistently refuse to accept the offer.

(33) Accepting feeling

For example:
"After all that no wonder you feel sad. If it were to happen to me I would feel that way too."

This is very similar to "reassurance" but technically is a reversal of the normal flow. In the language of psychiatry it is counter-transference rather than transference.

Two very curious behaviours occur as a result of the patient offering a criticism of some other agency, very often a hospital.

It would be wholly wrong to expect the GP to jump to the defence of other members of his profession. Judging by the sample of doctors examined here the probability of a doctor defending a hospital is exactly 50/50. More predictably, doctors will join patients in criticism of other parts of the health service. This pattern of behaviour is listed as below:

(34) Criticising other agencies

"I am often bewildered by what the Social Services departments think they are doing. If you have more trouble let me know."

This sort of criticism is very frequently heard after a referral or after the doctor has requested the help of a Social Service department. Occasionally a quite different type of criticism of another agency is heard. Its intent is very often to reinforce some sort of reassurance the doctor has given. The following is a good example:
"Now don't worry. Hospitals have got very odd views of hepatitis and they tend to frighten the patient without thinking. This is just another case of this happening."

The other side of the coin is the following:

(35) Justifying other agencies

For example:
"I think you can take it from me that hospitals know what they are doing"
or

"Nurses, you know, are highly trained people and are good at their job."

Justifying behaviours are much less frequent than critical behaviours. It is, again, largely a reaction to some complaint brought in by the patient. As the example in (34) above and the first example in (35) are provided by the same doctor, it seems that the doctor's view of the patient is more important than his view of the hospital.

There is also one interesting behaviour which occurs at various times in the consultation, which usually occurs when the doctor fears he might have offended the patient in some way.

(36) Apologising

A behaviour recorded primarily in the opening remarks made by the doctor as the patient enters the consulting-room.

For example:

"I am sorry that you have been kept waiting so long, please sit down"

or

"I am sorry to ask you to call in on a day like this, but the reports have just come back from the hospital and I thought we ought to discuss them."

Another form this takes is when a patient has returned from a referral and the doctor has to inform the patient that there is nothing wrong:

"Well, I'm very sorry to have to tell you that you made that journey for nothing,"

or it can preface bad news:

"Well, I'm sorry to have to tell you that the news is not good."

In a sense this latter form is very much a verbal cliché, but none the less the apologetic form is used. This sort of news is often broken in clichés anyway.

(37) Repeating what the patient has said for affirmation

For example:

"And you actually went to the child guidance clinic?"

or

"And you actually saw the consultant?"

Originally it was felt that these behaviours could be treated under the heading of "doubting". However, subsequent discussions with a number of the doctors indicates that there was no doubt at all in their mind. They said that they wished to make certain that the patient had actually said or done something. It occurs more frequently with immigrant patients than with British patients.

Occasionally it is very difficult to distinguish the repetition of patients' words from the two following behaviours.

(38) Chastising patients

For example:

"I wish you had come when all this started."

"Will you please wash before you come here."

"I think that is very silly of you."

Chastising is a comparatively rare behaviour and usually reflects a doctor's irritation with the way in which a patient appears to be behaving. Another cause of chastising can be the late introduction of a "by the way" offer from the patient. Where this behaviour has been observed, in all instances it has been possible to re-examine the doctor's feelings at the time. Most of the sample agreed that the behaviour is not particularly helpful, although it may help the doctor more than it does the patient. Most doctors claimed that the behaviour arose out of the stupidity of the patient and a consequent offence to the professional pride of the doctor. They also noted that the introduction of a "by the way" during a busy surgery is an extreme form of irritation.

(39) Challenging the patient

For example:
> "If you haven't been sleeping around again, how come you have got this condition?"

or
> "What do you mean you have not been taking those pills?"

Generally speaking, the outcome of a challenge from the doctor is observed to be a foregone conclusion, because most patients back down. However, this is not a general rule because some patients display a high level of aggression themselves. In the sample there also occurs one consultation in which a patient (who it appeared had a long history of hospitalisation for his psychopathic behaviour) responded to all challenges with overt aggression. Curiously the doctor in question rarely uses challenging behaviour in his normal consultations. Subsequent discussion with the doctor produced the information that he found the consultation hair-raising, and felt that his normally well controlled behaviour pattern vanished in the face of a direct confrontation.

This particular incident produced an insight into doctor behaviour which is rather more wide-ranging than simply dealing with a psychopath. Doctors can themselves provoke patient aggression quite unintentionally. Seven incidents were observed all involving extremely organically oriented doctors or extremely psychiatrically oriented doctors. In each incident the doctors concerned were facing a patient with a disorder which did not fit the doctor's preferences. As a result of the interaction between doctor and patient the patient in each case became more and more irritated. What was even more interesting was the way in which the doctor's preferred style also changed and became more and more authoritarian and dogmatic. At one stage one doctor actually said to his patient:
> "I will tell you what is wrong with you, I will tell you what your symptoms are and I will tell you what to do. I am the doctor here and you will kindly not forget that fact."

When this particular tape was replayed, this particular doctor, whilst he had clear memories of this patient, had no idea at all that he had become so dogmatic and overbearing.

CHAPTER 6

DOCTORS AND PATIENTS COPING WITH EACH OTHER: HOW THEY DO SO

In this section we propose to deal with the events which are part of the termination of the consultation. In the two previous sections we observed how a consultation starts and how it progressed to the point of diagnosis. A substantial number of consultations, whilst they have a greeting, move instantly to the point we are about to examine—because the diagnosis has already been made.

In Chapter 3 we observed that consultations appear to have a maximum of six phases. Many consultations run straight from Phase I to Phase IV. Phase IV, however, is never a certainty. For example, take the following consultation:

D. "Hello Mr Z——. Come in. Now then, you've just got back from Mr C——. Now then, I've got a letter here somewhere. Let me see. Ha ha. Mm, mm. Now then. Ah, yes. Well now. Nothing to worry about there. Good. Well now. Right ho. Ha, yes. Good. Take this to the chemist and get it made up. You will need to take the mixture twice a day. I would suggest before breakfast and before your evening meal. Then the tablets. Take those three times a day after meals."

P. "Did the specialist say I was all right?"

D. "Nothing at all there. All a false alarm. Now then. I want you back here in about a month. Okay. Good. How is Gladys getting on?"

P. "Oh, she's fine."

D. "Great stuff. Okay, then. See you then. Tell Marjorie on the way out will you. See you. 'Bye-bye."

In effect this doctor uses "reassurance" (see below) as a substitute for any real sharing of information with the patient. Even when pressed by the patient for some real information all that is given is more reassurance. This doctor also displays a style of moving quickly through the prescribing phase into termination.

There are also consultations in which final phases are reached within a few seconds. Take the following example:

D. "Come in. Hello. I'm Dr W——. Miss G——? Good. Now then, what can I do for you?"

P. "Well, I'm off to Egypt. . . ."

D. "To Egypt?"

P. "To Egypt. I need a smallpox injection and I was told by the travel agent to get a booster for my polio."

D. "Well, I think we can manage that. In fact we have some smallpox in the fridge. Hang on. I'll just make sure."

Twenty seconds silence.

D. "Here we are. Okay. Take your jacket off. Good. There we are. Now then. Your polio. What have you had in the past? Let's see. Oh, you have had a full course. That was six months ago. I think you will be okay. Are you going for very long?"

P. "No, only fifteen days."

D. "Oh, well, in that case you should have no problem."

P. "Somebody said I will need to have a jab against yellow fever."

D. "Yellow fever? Well you can if you wish. But I don't think you need it for Egypt. If you want that you will have to go into Birmingham. But I don't think you are going to dig a canal, are you?"

P. "Dig a canal?"

D. "Never mind. No. Don't worry about that. Is that all then? Good. Well, have a nice trip. Send me a card. 'Bye-bye."

In this consultation, once the doctor has gathered the travel information, there is no need for further diagnosis. He thus moves directly into the last two phases of the consultation.

On the whole very few consultations contain all six phases, but one phase which is not dependent upon the nature of the consultation is Phase IV. The majority of consultations studied (70 per cent) contain no real Phase IV of more than two seconds' duration. We are often, therefore, looking at consultations which run directly from the doctor making some sort of diagnostic decision to his starting the process of prescribing some future course of action.

The forms which Phase IV takes are comparatively limited when compared with any of the other phases, with the exception of Phases I and VI which are by definition idiosyncratic. In most cases, as already noted, Phase IV does not exist. There is also a form in which it has but a fleeting existence and is really little more than a form of conjunction used by the doctor to move from one part of the consultation (diagnostic) to another part (prescriptive).

(40) Summarising established positions to close off

For example:

"Now we know that you have difficulty climbing stairs, you have difficulty in getting to sleep, going to work in the morning tires you out, and that you have felt very run down for at least four months. In that case I think you ought to. . . ."

This summary by the doctor has been used to recapitulate what the patient has offered and is then used to move clearly into Phase V of the consultation, namely the detailing of treatment. A variation on this theme is the first person plural approach.

"Now then, let's see. Pains in the chest we have. Shooting pains behind the eyes we have. Blinding headaches and we are also having trouble with our waterworks. We don't look too good at all, do we?"

This type of Phase IV occurs very frequently with doctors who use "reassurance" (see below) as one of their main weapons. With both styles it is clear that the patient is expected to do no more than to agree with the doctor because there is no conversational space for the patient to occupy anyway.

Another fairly rapid transitional form is:

(41) Giving information or opinion

For example:

"I think you are suffering from. . . ."
"This condition is caused by. . . ."
"The medical name for this is. . . ."
"This can be cured by. . . ."

This behaviour is the commonest form of opening a consideration of the patient's condition, in which the initiative is taken by the doctor. Normally when it occurs it takes the form of a simple piece of medical information or an opinion. It is also usually fairly short in duration.

Both of these behaviours (40) and (41), however, do attempt to offer the patient a little insight into his condition. What is curious is that when one talks to doctors about this behaviour, most claim that they use it frequently. Yet on tape one finds that the majority switch quickly from Phase III to V with hardly a word to the patient *en route*. They only give the information as a prelude to termination in explanation of the nature of the prescription they are about to hand over.

(42) Reassuring

For example:

"I know how you feel, but don't worry about it."

"Everything is coming along nicely."

Reassurance is an interesting behaviour if only because the literature offers divided opinion on the subject. Sanhammer, Hays and Larson,[16] in their study of nurse behaviour, indicate that reassurance from the nurse is anything but reassuring. Equally a reading of Rogers[17] also leads to the conclusion that reassurance is not a particularly helpful device. On the other hand Hodson[18] seems supportive of the view that reassurance is one of the doctor's roles. Browne and Freeling[2] also appear to support reassurance as a function of the general practitioner. Further information about this issue might come from a research project into the credibility of various sources in which one might compare doctors with, for example, bank managers or accountants. There are several experiments indicating that the credibility of the source is a more important factor than what is said.[19] The doctor may well be in a position of greater credibility than the nurse. In the eyes of a patient it is probably true to say that if the doctor pronounces "You have not got X" then the patient will tend to believe he has not got X—if only because it fits in with the patient's desires. This cannot mean that everything a doctor says is accepted by every patient. Some patients are more sceptical of doctors than are others.

Reassurance, as such, may appear at any stage in the consultation. Its inclusion here is due to the fact that it occurs at this point more regularly than anywhere else, with the possible exception of the termination of the consultation. As many consultations really start at Phase IV, eg on-going treatment, returning referrals, it is not uncommon to find the doctor opening up the consultation with a piece of reassurance about the patient's condition.

(43) Predirectional probing

For example:

A. "If I were to say that you ought to go into hospital, how would you react?"

or

B. "If it is true that you are pregnant again, what would you want to do about it?"

This behaviour appears to be related to a doctor's uncertainty about the effect a prescription might have upon the patient. In the latter example, during discussion with the doctor, he rationalised his problems this way.

"The patient presented me with her symptoms and gave me the impression that she knew she was pregnant anyway. Thus my examination was simply confirming her fears. Six months previously she had enquired about 'family planning' but had reacted badly to the idea of 'birth control'. I subsequently discovered that she was a Roman Catholic, technically lapsed, but her husband and mother-in-law were still active communicants. Thus, my problem was simple. If she was there knowing herself to be pregnant and used that as the excuse to get in to see me, did she really come to talk

51

to me about an abortion? If she had religious difficulties over birth control how much more difficult would it be for her to face abortion."

This sort of probing then allows the doctor to explore possibilities almost at a hypothetical level, thus allowing himself and the patient to examine options, without actually being committed in advance to any of them.

Another example, and perhaps more common, is the following:

C. "How would you feel about changing your job?"

What is clear in each of the examples A, B and C is that the doctor has already made a diagnosis and has made some decisions about treatment. He is not sure, however, about the sort of response he is going to get from his patient and is sufficiently interested in his patient's feelings to seek out responses before committing himself to action.

(44) Summarising established positions to open up

For example:

"Well now, you seem to be feeling ill whenever you are alone or whenever you have to go to see your in-laws. Now what do you think this all means?"

The intention is quite unlike that in (51). Here the doctor is summarising what has been achieved in order to focus the patient's attention on an appreciation of his own problem. At this stage it seems as though the doctor wishes to prolong Phase IV rather than enter into the business of treatment.

This approach is by far the most obvious example of the fact that the doctor wishes the consultation to stay in Phase IV. Another much more overt example was provided by a doctor who was obsessed with the need to stop his patient's smoking.

D. "Now then. You have got all sorts of vague aches and pains in your chest. You have infections of the bronchus time and time again. You cough your heart out every morning. Every time you light up in the morning your heart starts to thump. I mean, apart from suggesting that we sit here waiting for a fall of soot, what should we talk about now?"

There is also some evidence that doctors will use this phase of the consultation when dealing with the problems of bereavement. This is quite interesting because the phase is used in this context by many GPs who never show any evidence of using it at any other time. The situation is fairly typical. Bereavement has clearly taken place some weeks before and the widow is in the process of being weaned off tranquillisers prescribed to help her cope with the situation. Whilst there is no typical form of words this sort of phrasing seems not untypical of the meaning:

"Now then, it's nearly seven weeks. You seem to be in quite good health yourself. I think that we ought to talk about the possibility of you giving up those tablets."

This doctor clearly is not yet in a position to prescribe a particular course of action, but he most certainly is clear about the course of action he would like to prescribe. He is not, however, wholly certain of the patient's ability to survive the course of action and is thus looking for her response.

(45) Using silence

This is well defined by Hayes et al[8] as "the absence of verbal communication". It is classified by them as a therapeutic technique, and in the context of the doctor/patient relationship retains that classification. It indicates that the doctor wishes the patient to do the talking and the thinking, and that the doctor is capable of controlling his urge to break silences. It is also used to slow down consultations and give both parties time to think. It might also sometimes cover the doctor's confusion as well as that of the patient.

We have already noted the fact that silence and listening are valuable techniques in Phase II. In Phase IV they serve a different purpose. What seems to be clear is that both doctor and patient know what the diagnosis is. They may also be aware of the prognosis. The doctor, however, does not wish to initiate the discussion but is leaving the patient to decide at what level the consultation is to restart. On the few occasions when this particular use of the behaviour was observed it was subsequently found that in each case the doctor either thought or knew that he was dealing with a terminal illness.

Phase V we have defined already as "detailing treatment or further investigation". This definition, of course, does not cover all the possible forms Phase V may take. For example, it may simply take the form of some advice as to the patient's future behaviour. Considerable numbers of patients, for example, seem to visit their GP for various inoculations prior to taking foreign holidays or business trips. The treatment is actually handed out in the surgery and Phase V may simply take a form such as follows:

> "Now then, let that have a couple of days and it should take"

or

> "Keep that clean now and it should be okay."

The most common form of Phase V is, in fact, a fairly straightforward direction.

(46) Directing

For example:

> "I want you to take this to the chemist. He will give you some tablets. These are to be taken three times daily, after meals"

or

> "I want you to take these tablets and come back to see me in a fortnight"

or

> "I will arrange for you to see Mr X. He is a specialist in the hospital. I will write to you telling you when an appointment has been made. After you have seen him come back and see me"

or

> "I want you to stop smoking, or at least start by cutting it down. When you have done that we will start some treatment."

These behaviours are common to most consultations. They are characterised by a clear directive to undertake some course of action, and this course of action is spelled out quite clearly. This type of behaviour is apparently well learned because in all but one instance it was clear and specific.

One real oddity, however, was observed:

> "Now there are enough tablets on that prescription to last you for a fortnight. I want you to take three a day, one after breakfast and one after the evening meal. Come back and see me in three weeks when the bottle is empty."

(47) Advising

For example:

"I think that you ought to take things a little easy for the next month or so. Then perhaps we might be able to do something more positive"

or

"If you take my advice, you will at least think about changing your job"

or

"I don't think that there is anything serious here. However, I think that I would like you to go on with the tablets for a week or so. Then, maybe it will clear up."

Advising appears to perform a similar function to directing. The distinction is that it lacks a positive act of direction and allows the patients some degree of latitude in how closely they adhere to whatever programme has been suggested.

(48) Seeking or accepting collaboration

This definition covers a range of behaviour in which the initiative might come from the doctor or from the patient. In its most obvious form one might well doubt whether the intention is collaborative or not.

"Well now, I think that we ought to work on this together."

This may well be another extension of the "royal we" favoured by so many doctors.

A slightly better example, again from an anti-smoking doctor, is the following:

"Now then, if you like, we will work together and try to sort this problem out."

In this case the insertion of "if you like" adds an element of patient choice to join in the contract or not to join in. On the whole, however, one must observe that patients are not apparently given to turning down such offers.

A much more obvious form of collaborating is the bargaining position taken again by anti-smoking doctors. In this example, as we shall see, a very clear contract is being spelled out:

"Well, if you are prepared to try to give up smoking, then I am prepared to try to do something about your chest."

There is also the end product of this type of relationship which can appear as follows:

"Well, you actually did go to see the dentist, so I will now try to treat the rest of you."

This latter example seems to appear in those situations where it is also apparent that the doctor has little sympathy for the patient.

Collaboration also can be initiated by the patient, as in the following example. The doctor has just completed spelling out a fairly complicated medical situation in which he has hinted at three or four different courses of treatment. His intention was clearly to test the patient reaction to each of these, but instead he earned the following;

"Well, doctor, what do you think we can do about it?"

To which he replied:

"Well I think, as you do, that we will have to work together."

Doctors appear to use collaborative approaches when they are facing difficult medical conditions or more particularly difficult patients. It has not been observed to be a primary strategy used by any of the doctors studied, but it does occur in a small number as an often used reserve strategy for any situation which does not seem to be going smoothly. Again, a large number of doctors seem to use it as a device for coping with smokers who have failed to take advice.

A tape provided by a private practitioner contains a remarkable response to the Budget of 1975, which placed yet another impost upon cigarettes.

D. "How many do you smoke a day?"

P. "Anything up to thirty."

D. "Come off it. I know you must get rid of at least two packs."

P. "Yes. Well, probably about forty-five."

D. "Good. Now then, you know and I know that you have got to give it up."

P. "Well, could I just cut down?"

D. "No. Give it up. It's not good for you. But I'll tell you what I'll do. Every morning you come in here and I will issue you with a packet of strong mints. You will pay me fifty pence for that privilege. If you then keep off cigarettes for twelve months, I will give you a one hundred and fifty pound holiday anywhere in the world. Right?"

P. "But that will cost you money."

D. "If you think that, then nicotine has befuddled you. In that case make it sixty-five pence."

P. "Well, okay. I'll tell you in the morning."

D. "Fine, I'll have your minties here."

Doctors do not seem to be very happy when patients offer collaboration, and many reject offers out of hand. Several members of the sample have expressed disapproval of patients who try to open up collaborative relationships. For these doctors, collaboration is a strategy which may very well be a demand for the doctor, but not for the patient. If time permits, and sufficient data comes to hand, then a separate investigation of collaborative strategies will be undertaken.

(49) Seeking out patient ideas

For example:
"Now what do you think you ought to do?"

or
"Next time this happens, what are you going to do then?"

A very common counselling behaviour in which the doctor is seeking to make sure that the patient has clearly decided to pursue some desirable course of action. It is also used in other situations such as family planning and abortion, where the ethic appears to be to place responsibility for decisions firmly upon the patient.

(50) Utilising patient ideas

Very often found in association with the above but not necessarily related. Doctors who have been on counselling programmes or who have read books on that subject have an almost stereo-typical form of words:
"Well now, if that is what you want to do, how do you think you will go about it?"

or
"If you do what you suggest in your first idea what do you think the problems will be?"

55

If the doctor is embarked upon a counselling approach to a patient then he will be utilising these particular behaviours before focusing the patient upon some final decision or other. In a more "normal" consultation the doctor may well be attempting a non-directive approach to some complex problem which is not amenable to authoritarian approaches.

(It may also be observed that if the doctor is using these last two behaviours, he will also be using a lot of encouragement and reflecting.)

Finally in this section we move to the ways in which a doctor actually gets a patient out of his consulting-room. In many ways this is a study of idiosyncrasies, as is the study of greeting patients. However, there are a number of styles which may be discerned and these are listed below.

(51) Symbolic termination (Weak)

The prime action here is not words but deeds. The most common indication of the fact that a consultation is over is the symbolic action of a piece of paper being torn from a pad of prescription forms. There are, of course, words to accompany this music but they are very secondary.

(52) Symbolic termination (Strong)

Some doctors use the socially learned technique of rising from their chairs and conducting the patient to the door. This is not a primary behaviour with more than 5 per cent but it is a very definite reserve behaviour for those who find that verbal cues and the above weak symbols have failed to move a patient.

(53) Direct verbal termination

For example:

"Right, off you go now. No need to worry. Come back and see me in a month"

or

"Come back and see me next week, will you? Make an appointment on the way out. All right? Cheerio."

This can be combined with (40) (above), in the following manner:

"Take this to the chemist, will you? And, oh, on your way out ask my secretary to come in."

There are other very rare terminations which have been observed to be rather more severe than any others:

"I do not wish to have you as a patient on my list. I will not prescribe those drugs for you. So please go away."

There are a variety of ways of closing consultations without being so direct. These have been labelled:

(54) Indirect verbal termination

For example:

"I suppose we have got as far as we can now. Don't you think so?"

This is really an invitation for the patient to leave unless there is still something on his mind.

This may also take the form of single words, in particular the word "well" posed in a questioning tone. It has the effect of causing some patients to close the consultation without any more being said.

(55) Patient termination

In very rare instances patients actually decided that the consultation was over. A few of these, as we shall see in the section on "dysfunctional consultations", are the result of terrible inter-personal problems between doctor and patient, but equally a few are quite genuine and satisfied closures which leave both parties quite content.

For example:

> "Well, I think I've got what I came for, doctor. I'll not use up any more of your time. Thanks a lot"

or

> "No, there's nothing else, doctor. Thank you very much. I'll be off now. See you next month. 'Bye-bye."

This latter is in response to a near standard preclosure behaviour of many doctors which is to pose the question:

> "Is there anything else?"

In 99 cases in 100 there is nothing and the patient is thus able to close. For the purposes of research the above statement would be classified as an indirect verbal termination.

CHAPTER 7

DOCTORS BEING NEGATIVE

The next section will deal specifically with those consultations which appear to be completely dysfunctional. This phenomenon occurs due to various and obvious circumstances and in particular due to communication problems with newly arrived immigrants. Equally, problems can occur if a patient deliberately chooses not to give the doctor some important information.

There are, however, consultations which do not appear to go wrong but in which the doctor appears to behave extremely negatively towards the patient. At one stage in the project a number of tapes were provided containing consultations between GPs and students demanding drugs. Whilst many of these consultations end in the patient being asked to leave without his drugs, the consultation cannot be regarded as a failure for the doctor.

For example:

D. "Come in. I'm Dr H——. Please sit down. What can I do for you?"

P. "Oh, I won't take long. I'm normally Dr G——'s patient. He prescribes these for me."

D. "Dr G——?"

P. "Yes, you know, in the university doctor's place."

D. "But this practice is nothing to do with that one."

P. "Oh, yes, I know. But he said if he was not on I should come here."

D. "What for?"

P. "Well, for a supply of these."

D. "Do you know what these are?"

P. "Well, yes, you see I'm very run down and cannot face the exams. These help, you know."

D. "They do not help you to do anything but become more useless."

P. "Well, I have to have them. You must give them to me."

D. "I do not have to give you anything. I will not give you a prescription for anything like this."

P. "But what bloody use are doctors if they won't give you the prescriptions. I've got my rights, you know."

D. "You can take your rights along with this empty bottle and walk back to where you came from."

P. "Won't you give me some amytol then?"

D. "No. I will not give you anything. Not even an aspirin."

P. "I'll commit suicide."

D. "Well go and do it outside. Clear off."

P. "I will. I will. I'll take aspirins."

D. "Well make sure you take at least one hundred and fifty. Now clear off."

P. "I'll tell Dr G—— you refused me."

D. "When I see Dr G—— I may have some questions to ask him about you. Now stop wasting my time and go. If you don't I will have you put out."

In this consultation the doctor adopts a fairly negative approach to the patient early on. As a doctor he has strong views on drug dependence and drug users and is quite unlikely to allow himself to be manipulated by the patient. Examining his behaviour proved valuable because once he has discovered why this patient is there he starts to use a behaviour pattern which, to date, has not been described in this study. His behaviour can be explained up to the point where he says:

"They do not help you to do anything but become more useless"
in the following manner:

(a) Offering of self. Broad opening.
(b) Repeating what the patient said for affirmation.
(c) Giving information.
(d) Direct question.
(e) Direct question (or if he already suspects it is a challenge).

It is very difficult to describe the above quotation with any of the terms we have developed to date. It is not really "giving information or opinion". What he is in fact doing is rejecting the last thing the patient said.

About 3 per cent of the consultations studied contained substantial elements of this sort of negative behaviour, although many more consultations contained small quantities of negative behaviour, especially in response to patient initiatives which were not appreciated by the doctor.

Eight broad categories of negative behaviour were defined although this may well not be a very exhaustive list.

N1 Rejecting patient offers

For example:

P. "By the way, doctor, do you think I ought to have mentioned these headaches?"

D. "We'll talk about that next time"

or

P. "What on earth am I going to do about him, doctor?"

D. "Let's concentrate upon your rash, shall we, and leave that to another time."

In these examples the patient is making an attempt to introduce into the consultation new material. The material may or may not be relevant to the consultation, although it must be of some importance to the patient. In these instances the doctor is making a decision to limit the content of the consultation and therefore decides to reject the new material offered by the patient. Some doctors are extraordinarily sensitive about their role or status. They show this by a curious form of behaviour which can do nothing but drive home to the patient that doctors are doctors and as such superior to patients.

N2 Reinforcing self-position

For example:

"Now I think that I know what is best for you"

or

"I am the doctor and I will do whatever prescribing needs to be done."

Sometimes the doctor is irritated by some remark or some behaviour of the patient and will react in this fashion in an attempt to assert some sort of dominance over the patient. A very frequent cause of this sort of irritation in some doctors is the self-prescribing patient who is given to asking for specific quantities of specific drugs. Occasionally it can also be caused by doctors being insufficiently sensitive to the needs of the patient and misunderstanding what the patient is trying to say. There are many occasions when doctors are confronted by problems of such complexity that they seem to be as helpless as the patient. One reasonable reaction is at least to appear to be in control, and this may be achieved by asserting the self.

N3 Denying patient

For example:

"I do not wish to have you on my list"

or

"I am not interested in what you have to say to me."

The two examples above are derived from interviews between drug addicts and doctors who have fears of becoming recognised as "drug prescribers". Such behaviour is, of necessity, emphatically negative. The denying behaviour may well be less forcefully applied, simply by ignoring most of what the patient says.

Denying may also take the form of a frequent "shut out". In some consultations it may be noted that the doctor will stop the patient when he has heard what he wishes to hear. He will interrupt a patient, thus stopping any further flow, and asks quite a different question. The cumulative effect of this is to deny the patient an opportunity to speak. It need not, therefore, be a single behaviour but the cumulative effect of several.

N4 Refusing patient ideas

For example:

"No, I don't think that will help at all"

or

"That sort of approach will get you nowhere at all."

Some patients do occasionally offer ideas of what their treatment ought to be. Doctors who frequently use "encouraging" also are noted as "seeking patient ideas" and "using patient ideas". Some patients produce ideas whether the doctor encourages or not and the doctor then has a choice whether to use these ideas or not. It has been observed that in some situations doctors become extremely irritated when patients offer ideas, and not only are the ideas refused but one also observes that this is followed by some sort of reinforcing of the doctor's position.

N5 Evading patient questions

For example:

P. "Is it serious, doctor?"

D. "Well, let's talk about your diet"

or

P. "Am I going to be able to go back to work?"

D. "Let's not worry about that at the moment, let's consider the treatment."

There are often very good and sound reasons for evading a patient's question. Many doctors, for example, in life-threatening and in terminal cases will never admit the truth to a patient unless severely pressed. There are also instances when patients demand answers to questions which the doctor himself does not understand. Many patients offer doctors very limited insights into personal problems and then ask him to make a snap decision on the basis of what he has been offered. Very frequently this will be part of a manipulative strategy of husband against wife or vice versa or mother against child. The doctor is seen here as a useful ally who has to be won over as soon as possible.

There are also instances in which doctors evade questions because the question itself is a nuisance. Patients often ask questions about events which take place earlier in the consultation and some doctors find this an irritation. They will therefore use some form of evasion to conceal their irritation and avoid answering the question.

N6 Not listening

There are occasional pieces of evidence which indicate that the doctor is not listening. Some doctors admit that there are patients who regularly come with the same or different complaints, and who are so irritating that the best defence is not to listen. The same doctors admit that they also have occasional anxieties that they might have missed something of importance.

Not listening is also a very soft form of the "shut out". The only difference is that the non-listening doctor is usually not prepared to interrupt a patient.

A number of doctors make noises whilst not listening. This is a very common habit, particularly when the doctor is writing out a prescription. Occasionally, however, the patient will offer some totally new information during this time which has absolutely no effect at all on the doctor. Subsequent replay of the tape produces a range of reaction from anger to severe anxiety.

N7 Refusing to respond to feeling

For example:

"Oh, I do feel badly about the whole thing, doctor."

"Well, take your tablets."

Patients sometimes offer doctors insights into their emotional state which are very useful to the doctor. Some doctors, however, do not like too much of this type of behaviour and try hard to stop the flow. In the example above the doctor makes a statement which does not match the emotionality of what the patient has said.

N8 Confused noise

There is one constant characteristic of all consultations which are not working well. It is normally observed as a situation in which both patient and doctor are talking at the same time and neither stops in order to listen to what the other is saying.

All of these behaviours are described as being negative. Many of them are also counter-productive on most occasions. This does not mean that they are necessarily bad—indeed the reverse might well be true. There is also the point that doctors, to some extent, have to be protected against patients, and to this end negative behaviour is very useful.

CHAPTER 8

CONSULTATIONS WHICH GO WRONG

During the study a number of consultations caused a lot of interest because much of what was recorded apparently made no sense. It was not due to any foreign language being spoken, or indeed to any medical mysteries. It was quite simply that doctor and patient appeared to be having quite separate consultations.

In one of the very first tapes studied the following interaction was recorded as part of a consultation which in every other respect was quite normal. The excerpt itself began without any warning after the doctor had examined the patient subsequent to her offering pains in the chest as a symptom. She also made apparent that the pains had started during the night.

D. "What time did the pain start?"

P. "I saw him at three or four in the afternoon . . . but he didn't seem to notice me then. . . ."

D. "Yes, but what time did it start?"

P. "There was nothing to be said. Nothing at all [Crying]. I wasn't there at first. It didn't seem real."

D. "What?"

P. "When I came home."

D. "At what time did it . . . ?"

P. "It started at nine."

D. "The pains started at nine?"

P. "What pains?"

D. "The ones you said you had last night."

P. "I'm not talking about them."

D. "Oh. I was asking you what time they came on."

In this excerpt the patient is clearly not listening to the question which the doctor keeps asking. The patient is also telling him things other than that which he wishes to hear.

This particular consultation returned quickly to a more normal (and hopefully fruitful) form of communication. The short excerpt, however, stands out as a totally odd occurrence which seems to relate to nothing at all in that consultation. Such events, if not quite so dramatic, do occur occasionally in consultations and in most instances the doctor or the patient refocuses the consultation. There are occasional consultations in which such a pattern of mis-communication may well go on for two or three minutes.

Then there are other consultations in which it is clear that the matters which have never been discussed are of more significance than those matters which have been discussed. There are also occasional consultations in which things said by one party do not seem to be heard by the other party.

All of these phenomena produce a small number of consultations in which doctor and patient find themselves seeking to achieve goals which are not shared or even understood by the other party. When the parties remain in ignorance of each other's goals the consultation seems to drag inexorably into failure. By any definition these consultations are dysfunctional.

In order to establish what could constitute criteria which might define dysfunction, certain statements were tested upon individuals and groups and out of these arose a sequence of statements which enable one to hazard a defini-tion:

(*a*) A consultation between a doctor and a patient is a goal-seeking activity in which both parties may have goals.

(*b*) The goals of the consultation may be differently perceived by the doctor and by the patient.

(*c*) A consultation may be described as wholly successful when both parties come to an agreement upon the goals of the consultation and achieve these to their own satisfaction.

(*d*) A consultation may also be successful when both parties to the consul-tation perceive each other's goals whilst only one party achieves its goal.

(*e*) A consultation may be successful when only one party is aware of the goals and achieves them.

(*f*) A consultation may be dysfunctional when both parties appear to fail:
  (i) to comprehend each other's goals and
  (ii) to achieve either set of goals.

These statements create a spectrum of consultations which range from the wholly successful (in terms of goals and achievements) through partly successful (in terms of one party or the other achieving goals) to the situation in which neither party appears to achieve anything. Thus a consultation in which the doctor achieves his goals, but does not achieve the patient's goals, would not be regarded as dysfunctional. A good example of this is contained in a consultation involving a patient returning to the doctor for a repeat prescription. This particular doctor made a habit of always undertaking a repeat examination before issuing a repeat prescription. In one instance the patient, reluctantly, underwent the examination. The result revealed a totally new set of symptoms for which the management was hospitalisation rather than the expected repeat chemotherapy. In this situation the doctor achieved his goal, which might be described as appropriate treatment for observed symptoms. The patient, who had the goal of collecting a repeat prescription, did not achieve it.

Such an example, whilst not common, is typical of a number of consultations and may be said to reflect the strength of the doctor's position in the consultation. There are also cases in which quite the reverse occurs, when patients manipulate doctors into doing things they might not wish to do.

In the research project we were able to identify 37 consultations in which it appeared that there was no congruence of goals and there appeared to be no satisfied party at the outcome. There also appeared to be a clear degree of inter-actional confusion because many of the statements or questions made by the doctor bear no relationship to the apparent responses made by the patient, and vice versa. It was also possible to check the content of 18 of these consultations with the doctors concerned, and in all but one case consultation was agreed on as being dysfunctional. One other consultation, not included in the 37, is interesting because it highlights so many of the characteristics of dysfunction. In the transcript which follows, a behavioural interpretation of the doctor's remarks is offered.

To set the scene for this consultation it must be pointed out that the doctor in question knew the patient very well and judged by her record she well merits his description as "a nuisance". The doctor himself is very much oriented towards organic concepts of illness, taking the view that his prime task is to eliminate all possible organic causes of illness before searching out psychosomatic causes.

Given this particular situation, and the fact that this happened to be a fairly busy surgery, one can see how the first half of this consultation drifts into severe dysfunction.

D. "Good afternoon, and what is it you've come to see me about?" (Broad question.)

P. "It's me eyes, actually."

D. "Your eyes . . .?" (Repeating for affirmation.)

P. "They're itching, smarting. . . ."

D. "How long have they been doing that?" (Placing events in time.)

P. "Oh . . . coming on for a week now. . . . I don't know whether it's the worry, but Paul. . . ."

D. (Interrupting.) "Have you been using any make-up?" (Direct question.)

P. "No, I don't use make-up. . . ."

D. ". . . because that is a very common. . . ."

P. "No, I don't use make-up. . . ."

D. ". . . cause of this sort of thing." (Giving information.)

P. "I had this once before in . . . about . . . three or four years ago when I had an emotional upset. . . . So it could be that."

At this point both talk at once, and the doctor appears to be dismissing the emotional cause of the itch (rejecting patient offer). The patient keeps repeating "but the itch . . . but the itch".

D. "All right, I'll give you some ointment to put on them which will stop it from itching and burning." (Directing/giving information.)

P. "Oh, do you know, doctor, I don't know what . . . that Paul has got himself into. . . ."

(At this point the consultation was interrupted by another patient entering the consulting-room in error.)

P. ". . . he's gone and got himself picked up by the police last Sunday night . . . attempted robbery . . . he had this big screwdriver with him. If that isn't bad enough, it's cost me fifteen pounds to get them out of me house up in Bury, and thirty pounds for me husband. The place is in a . . . it's been

absolutely vandalised . . . the garden's like a rubbish dump. The garage . . .
I'm not joking . . . I was up there. . . ."

D. "Where, in Thomas Street?" (Clarifying.)

P. "No, in Bury. I'm not there now. . . ."

D. "Oh . . . er." (Indicating understanding.)

P. "I'm getting it back. I couldn't go back and look at the damage and
vandalism they've done to a beautiful house like that. It's lost me five
hundred pounds off the price of it. So I'll just have to take four. The income
tax man says I may be liable but . . . capital gains tax on the . . . sale of it.
Whether I'm buying property on the . . . with the money or not . . . there's
no way round it. I couldn't stay up there on me own . . . with those horrible
neighbours. I'd just go to pot again."

D. "Well, go and get this ointment and put a little of it along the eyelids three
times a day." (Directing and summarising to close off.)

This attempt to finish the consultation failed completely and the patient
continued to talk, unaware of the irritation she caused the doctor.

P. "What would you do with him, doctor? He needs psychiatric help . . . I'm
positive . . . I really am, doctor . . . the things he does. . . ."

D. "Well, maybe he does act in a peculiar way." (Reassurance.)

Confused noise.

D. ". . . he acts in something like a rather anti-social way, and I'm not sure
that he does need psychiatric help. . . ." (Reassurance.)

P. "He went away and I didn't know where he was for a month . . . at that
festival . . . I had to get the police to look for him. . . ."

D. (Interrupting.) "How old is he now?" (Direct question.)

P. "He's nearly eighteen, doctor . . . he's muffed the. . . ."

D. "When is he eighteen?" (Direct question.)

P. "February the tenth . . . he's muffed the college up."

D. "I'm afraid it's likely that he's going to get into various scrapes from time
to time. . . ." (Summarising to close off.)

Short confused noise.

D. ". . . and the best thing you can do is to cut your losses . . . I don't think
that you are going to be able to influence him one way or another." (Summary continued.)

P. "But when he's with me he is normal and happy and quiet and there's
not an argument between the two of us . . . doing these stupid things. Yet
when he's with me he doesn't do these things. . . ."

D. "No." (Doubting.)

Short confused noise in which both are talking and neither is listening.

D. "He has always been erratic. . . ."

P. "But he. . . ."

D. "Maybe he is psychiatric. . . ."

P. "He's not been right since his father died. . . ."

As far as possible the content of confused noise is recorded here.

There follows 30 seconds of confused noise in which the doctor is trying to
ask some questions and the patient is still trying to tell the doctor how well
behaved the boy was. Then for a short while the consultation drifts into what
sounds like a discussion, but in fact is nothing more than two people talking to
themselves, alternately.

64

D. "He has been in trouble between the ages of eleven and eighteen you know. . . ."

P. ". . . and at school they used to upset him by saying all sorts of things about his father being dead. . . ."

D. ". . . and as long as I've known him he has never been one hundred per cent perfect as you might say. . . ."

P. ". . . I do think that. . . ."

D. ". . . he isn't. . . ."

Three more seconds of confused noise before the doctor manages to get a question across to the patient.

D. "How many times has he been in court?" (Direct question.)

P. "This is the first time for. . . ."

D. "No, but how many times has he been in court?" (Direct question.)

P. "Three times."

D. "Three times now." (Repeating for affirmation.)

More confused noise.

The consultation concludes with an unhappy woman leaving the surgery carrying a prescription which may solve the problem of the rash on her eyelids.

A number of observations may be made about this consultation. The first is that the patient is "playing the patient game", or, in Balint's terms, using some symptoms as an excuse to get into the consulting-room. She had no real intention of talking about her rash except as a symptom of something else. The doctor, clearly wishing to move this consultation quickly, accepts the offer of a rash but is left holding it when the patient starts to talk about concerns more real to her at that moment.

Secondly, this consultation like most dysfunctional consultations is full of confused noise, in which both parties appear to be talking and neither seems to be listening. It may well be possible in this case, and in several others, that neither wishes to listen to what the other has to say.

Thirdly, there is a conflict of objectives and an almost total lack of opportunity to achieve what either party may want. The doctor clearly wishes to conclude this consultation quickly whilst the patient appears to want some sort of support in her problems. (What is also not clear here is that the young man she refers to is not this doctor's patient.) The doctor does in fact finally get her out, but has used up nearly 11 minutes of valuable time in the process. In that he did finally get the patient out of his consulting-room, he may be seen as having achieved some sort of objective.

A totally different sort of dysfunction is demonstrated in the next example. The consultation drifts into dysfunction almost as soon as it begins.

D. "Come in. Good morning Mrs G——. I don't think we have met before."

P. "Yes, we have. I came to see you three years ago and you gave me some tablets."

D. "Are you sure you came to me?"

P. "Yes, you are Dr P——, are you not?"

D. "Yes, I am, but I don't seem to have any records. Would you please hold on a minute whilst I talk to my receptionist?"

(There follows a short telephone conversation with the receptionist which produces no result.)

65

D. "Anyway, I am sorry, Mrs G——. Now then, what is it today?"
P. "Well, I've got this pain again."
D. "Which pain?"
P. "The pain I had last time I came in."
D. "Oh, I see."
P. "What?"
D. "The pain—go on, tell me about it."
P. "I thought all doctors were supposed to keep records."
D. "Well, of course we do. I can't think how yours has come to have gone astray."
P. "Well, I don't like the idea of my records being lost somewhere."
D. "Well, I assure you that it must be here somewhere. Please don't worry about it. It will turn up, you know."
P. "Hmm. Well, I don't like it. I think I would like to see another doctor."
D. "But Mrs G——."

At this point the patient got up and left the room.

This terribly unfortunate situation left the doctor quite helpless. Equally, the patient had managed to do nothing except upset herself and a doctor. A discussion with the doctor in question confirmed that the patient was in a highly anxious condition when she came in, and this may well have been aggravated by the loss of a piece of paper. The patient did not return to the doctor in question, nor did she return to any other member of his practice.

In the first half of the research project a count was made of the number of times records went astray or were mixed up. Out of 969 consultations 59 instances of lost or wrong records were noted. (This figure may well be greater but no evidence exists on tape.) This is the only instance of a patient taking umbrage at the matter. It is, however, a case in which neither the patient nor the doctor achieved anything.

The next example consultation is not classified under the heading "dysfunctional" even though the doctor concerned, after listening to the recording, considered it to be so. It is, in fact, an example of a consultation in which one party appears to partially gain its objectives whilst the other party gains nothing.

In this case the patient is female, aged about 45 to 50 and social class D. She made an appointment in an evening surgery which started around 4.45 pm. So far the doctor has seen nine patients and is averaging 3·4 minutes per consultation. His last two patients, however, last for seven and eight minutes, and six patients are now waiting in the waiting-room.

D. "Come in. How are you today? Do sit down. What can I do for you?" (i)
P. "Can I have a certificate, please?"
D. "For what?" (ii)
P. "Like last time, for work."
D. "I thought we said that you were going to go back to work at the end of last week. Have you been off all this week as well?" (iii)
P. "Oh. I don't want to go back."
D. "But you should go back to work. You know as well as I do that you only sit around the house and worry and do nothing. It does you no good at all. You really must go back to work. You were quite all right until about a few weeks ago. Then you came in and you were telling me about how tired you were, and how you needed a rest. Now you've had a rest, you've had some

treatment. I am sure there is nothing wrong with you at all. And now you say you've been off all this week as well." (iv)

P. "Oh, I get so fed-up every time I think of going back to that place."

D. "Well, you must face up to it, you know. I think it will do you a lot of good to get back to work." (v)

P. "But I can't go back this week. I need a little more rest before I go. I've been off now for three days this week. So I can't go back until next week now. So I've got to have a certificate or I'll not get what's coming."

D. "So you are going back next week then?" (vi)

P. "Oh, yes. If I feel well next Monday, I'll go back."

D. "Well, I'll write this for you now. But you must go back next week." (vii)

P. "Oh, yes, doctor. 'Bye-bye. Oh, can I have the prescription too?"

D. "Now you do not need anything at all this time." (viii)

P. "But I'll be lost without those pills."

D. "No. In my opinion you do not need them at all." (ix)

P. "But can't I have them just this week?"

D. "No. There is no way at all that I could justify that to myself. Now off you go. Let's have no more of this." (x)

This consultation is comparatively short and appears to have very little about it which is satisfactory. The doctor in question volunteered some more information. It appears that the same patient turned up in his partner's surgery the next day, asking for her prescription "which the doctor forgot to give me yesterday". The partner obliged; an action which caused a little friction in the practice on the following day.

If we examine the consultation in terms of possible objectives we might well hypothesise that the patient had two possible objectives which were made manifest to the doctor. Firstly, she wanted to clear herself for another week away from work (objective achieved) but she also wished to collect another prescription (not achieved in her first consultation).

Other doctors, and indeed the doctor in question, have commented upon one feature of the consultation which has a lot of significance in terms of concealed objectives. It seems as though the patient made two attempts to talk to the doctor about her feelings concerning her work (see units (iii) and (iv)).

If we examine this consultation in terms of its phases we can see that it contains a Phase I (relating to the patient) and a very brief Phase II. It is, however, very difficult to argue that Phase II is in any way complete. If we accept the interpretation that this patient had a desire to talk about her feelings concerning her place of work then it has not got off the ground. The consultation then moves rapidly into Phases V and VI. The request for a prescription is a concealed "by the way", which fails to produce any results.

In terms of behaviour items the consultation may be interpreted as follows:

(i) Recognition. Broad opening. Directing. Broad opening.
(ii) Direct question.
(iii) Chastises patient.
(iv) Giving advice. Chastising. Directing. Giving information. Giving opinion. Chastising.
(v) Offering opinion.
(vi) Seeking patient ideas.
(vii) Summarising to close off.

67

    (viii) Rejecting patient offers.

    (ix) Denying patient.

    (x) Justifying self. Directing. Chastising.

The doctor, when questioned about this interview, did admit that he was extremely irritated by the patient, but was quite unable to explain the real source of his irritation. He suggested that it might have been due to the fact that she had not returned to work and thus completed a treatment which he thought ought to have been completed. He also considered that it might have been due to his need to complete his surgery on time, but on listening to the complete tape, he considered this unlikely. What he did admit to is significant. He claimed that on listening to the tape, he realised that he had made his mind up as soon as the patient declared she had not returned to work. He was then determined to get her to return. He lost sight of this objective as soon as he had given her a certificate and was then extremely angry with himself when she asked for her prescription. As in the case of the last example, it is clear than an interview with the doctor concerned is often important to the understanding of the consultation itself. In this particular case the doctor was available for such an interview and decided that by his own standards this particular case really ought to be listed under the heading of dysfunctional. It is, however, a good example of a patient achieving her objectives at the expense of the doctor.

In the study of dysfunctional consultations, 37 consultations were found which were very clearly cases of dysfunction. These were drawn from the then total of 963 consultations available. (Subsequently a further 1151 consultations were submitted and the overall incidence of certain dysfunction drops to 56 in 2114.)

Of the 37 studied:

    26 occurred during evening surgeries

    1 during an afternoon ante-natal examination

    9 during morning surgery

    1 could not be placed in time by the doctor and there was no indication on the tape.

The first test concerned the degree to which the incidence of the dysfunctional consultations reflects the actual time structure of the total sample:

    495 consultations take place during the evening surgery

    103 consultations take place in the afternoon

    314 take place in the morning

    27 could not be accurately placed in time.

This appears to indicate that there is a much higher probability of dysfunction occurring during the evening. However, as the sample of consultations is not based upon any time analysis, and as practices have a great variation of time in the structure of a day's work, this part of the data serves only as an indication for further enquiry.

Several doctors were asked about the relative pressures upon them to complete a surgery, and here again the evidence is very mixed. Some doctors appeared to react more to the stress of ending a morning surgery, in order to visit patients, whilst others reacted more to the idea of completing an evening surgery in order to get home:

    20 occur with female patients

11 occur with male patients

   6 occur with parent/child consultations.

In terms of the balance of sexes there is a better correlation:

Consultations with female patients	380
Consultations with male patients	225
Consultations with parent/child	198
Consultations with male/female	77
Consultations with family and other groups	59*

The 37 clearly defined dysfunctional consultations were compared with a random sample of equal size drawn from the total number of consultations available. After the 37 had been eliminated a sample in excess of 900 was left. These consultations range from those where there was an ideal congruence of objectives to those consultations in which one party or the other achieves its goals alone. We are thus comparing dysfunctional, according to our definitions, with "not dysfunctional".

It must be noted at this point that this is not necessarily a comparison of "good" and "bad". Whilst doctors may regret a dysfunctional consultation one cannot describe the event as being bad. Many doctors have argued that if the word "bad" is to be applied to consultations it must be applied to those consultations in which doctors appear to diagnose illnesses in the absence of any information, or those in which patients manipulate doctors to some end which is neither medically nor socially desirable.

The first component of the consultation measured in the two samples concerned is "confused noise". All clearly distinguishable doctor's speech was measured for duration. Then all patient speech was measured. Also measured was the amount of time in which neither party spoke and the amount of time in which all parties were speaking at the same time (confused noise). The results are as follows:

	Dysfunctional	Not dysfunctional
Doctor noise	29%	23%
Patient noise	38%	51%
Silence	7%	16%
Confused noise	26%	10%

A very severe test was applied to the confused noise. Any occasion upon which both parties appeared to be talking simultaneously was classified as "confused noise". In a number of cases what each party is saying is easily decipherable, but for those concerned it is assumed that they were unable to hear each other because they were talking.

There are a number of features here which are worthy of comment. Most significant is the difference in the actual proportions of "confused noise". It has already been noted that dysfunctional consultations appear to suffer from a considerable amount of confused noise, and this data demonstrates that its

---

*The majority of this group are consultations between doctors and non-English-speaking immigrants, members of their families and, occasionally, interpreters. These consultations are extremely difficult to assess because, due to cultural differences, most of the patients from the Indian sub-continent appear very willing to accept anything the doctor may say. There are two instances in which the doctor discovers that he is examining the wrong patient, but as the error was subsequently rectified, these instances cannot be regarded as dysfunctional.

incidence is two-and-a-half times that which occurs in "non-dysfunctional" consultations. Ascribing blame for this, or simply seeking causes, it does seem that it is more frequently caused by doctors trying to interrupt patients than by any other cause. Discussions with doctors concerning their own dysfunctional consultations have produced a number of insights.

In most cases it is true to say that doctors do realise that something is going wrong during the consultation. Recognising this, they then try to take hold of events by talking. The patient, however, does not accept the cue to stop and continues talking—thus dragging the consultation further into dysfunction.

Another interesting explanation was offered as follows: The patient comes in and knows that she is going to say all sorts of things to the doctor but does not know how to start. So she offers a symptom, preferably one she has offered on several occasions before. Then as soon as she makes this offer, the doctor, who already suspects the worst, seizes the symptom and starts to treat it. The patient, however, realises what has happened and starts to offer the real causes of her attendance for fear of not having them heard. In order to find out that this is happening one of them has got to stop. Then it becomes a game of "chicken".

The other interesting feature in this set of data is the fact that the amount of silence in dysfunctional consultations is so much less. Silence was measured by collecting together all the parts of a consultation in which no one was speaking. It might occur as a result of a question, or it might well occur whilst someone is talking and just stops momentarily to think. There is also an interesting relationship between the quantity of silence and the quantity of confused noise. Consultations which drift into dysfunction often change in this respect. The quantity of silence decreases and the quantity of confused noise increases.

The 37 clearly dysfunctional consultations were compared with a random sample of "non-dysfunctional" consultations. The purpose of the comparisons was to discover whether there are significant differences in the various time allocations within consultations and whether the total time spent in dysfunctional consultations was less or more than in non-dysfunctional consultations.

Apart from the overall length of a consultation, the amount of time spent in Phase II and the amount of time spent in Phase IV was measured. The reasons for the selection of these two phases are as follows:

1. Phase II is when the doctor finds out why the patient is there. If this is cut short then the doctor runs the risk of making assumptions about the patient which may not be shared by the patient.

2. Phase IV is a point in the consultation where the sharing of information might allow both parties to discover what is going wrong with the consultation (assuming that anything is wrong).

3. Phases I and VI are so idiosyncratic that any measure would be meaningless.

4. Phase III is a matter of medical judgement upon which the researcher is not qualified to comment.

5. Phase V is so late in the consultation that in many cases it fails to occur in a dysfunctional consultation. It is also used by doctors to stop a dysfunctional consultation and can become inseparably confused with Phase VI.

Test A

A comparison of average consultation times

The data was analysed using the t-test for independent samples where population variances are different. This is a test of the significance of the difference in the observed means.

	Dysfunctional	Non-dysfunctional
Mean of Sample	4·14	5·31
Variance of Sample	1·89	6·92

(Consultation times were recorded in minutes.)

The excess of $5·31-4·14 = 1·17$ minutes of the non-dysfunctional mean over the dysfunctional mean has a statistical significance of 1 per cent (approx), ie if both population means were the same such an excess would occur in about one such investigation out of a hundred. Thus we can say that the data reveals that the mean time for a non-dysfunctional consultation is higher than that for a dysfunctional consultation.

Note the difference in sample variance for the two types of consultation. The distribution of times for the non-dysfunctional consultations has not only a higher mean but also a much higher variance. This greater variability of the non-dysfunctional data is reflected in the data ranges, ie greatest/least observation in each set of data.

Data Ranges (in minutes)

	Least	Greatest	Range
Dysfunctional	2·10	8·20	6·10
Non-dysfunctional	1·55	14·80	13·25

The difference in distributional spreads is quite marked for the higher times: only 6 out of 36 dysfunctional consultations are longer than 6 minutes, while 15 out of 39 non-dysfunctional consultations have this property.

Several doctors have commented that when they find themselves involved in some degree of dysfunction they find that time seems to pass very slowly. As a result of this feeling they believed that dysfunctional consultations lasted much longer than any other sort of consultation.

What they may well be indicating is that they find themselves in dysfunctional consultations which they subsequently correct. If that is so then in this set of tests they would be listed as "non-dysfunctional".

One observation may be made about wholly dysfunctional consultations. Doctors realising they are in some sort of trouble use all sorts of devices to end the consultation. One doctor admitted that he wrote a prescription for a placebo and took the patient to the door whilst she was still talking. Others relate to a single symptom and seek to treat that alone. The effect of this is to shorten the normal pattern of closure. Sometimes it takes three or four attempts to finish off a consultation, and in these cases the doctor may be heard saying the same things over and over again until he finally manages to get the patient out of the room. To some extent this is substantiated by the much narrower range of times shown by the dysfunctional consultation.

Proportion of time spent on Phase II

Once again, an independent samples t-test (this time equal variances were assumed) was used to test the difference in mean proportions. Both sets of

71

data exhibit quite marked positive skew which reduces the reliability of the test; nevertheless it is still a useful exercise since lack of normality is not so serious in large samples.

	Dysfunctional	Non-dysfunctional
Mean of Sample	0·139	0·252
Variance of Sample	0·016	0·026

Although the two sample variances, 0·016 and 0·026, appear to be different, a variance ratio test showed that the population variances can be regarded as the same.

The difference in means $0·252 - 0·139 = 0·113$ is significant at the 1 per cent level on a one-tailed test (ie if the means were really the same, such an experimental result would be obtained only on one occasion in a hundred). Thus we conclude that the average proportion of time spent on Phase II is greater for non-dysfunctional consultations.

Proportion of time spent on Phase IV

Both sets of data exhibit very strong positive skew (much more than the Phase II data analysed above). Zero proportions—non-occurrence of Phase IV—are prominent in both sets. On each set over half the observations are less than or equal to 0·05 and in addition both sets have extremely long tails—reaching 0·39 for dysfunctional and 0·29 for non-dysfunctional.

Because of the heavily skewed nature of the data, a non-parametric test, the Wilcoxon Rank Sum Test, was used instead of a t-test. The result of this test leads to the conclusion that the two sets of data have the same distribution; thus as regards Phase IV proportions there is no difference between dysfunctional and non-dysfunctional.

This data goes a long way to emphasising the importance of Phase II of the consultation. As we can see, non-dysfunctional consultations contain a greater proportion of Phase II than the dysfunctional consultations. Naturally, in this data there are many consultations in which Phase II occurs more than once. Some doctors are sensitive to the fact that the first symptom they sought to treat is not the real basis of the patient problem. None the less it is necessary to repeat a point made earlier on. If the doctor is certain that he knows why the patient is there he will often find that he is not dealing with the first offer made by the patient. It would also seem to be common sense to make as accurate a diagnosis as possible to provide the most efficacious treatment—thus hopefully reducing the number of times a patient will return.

Non-dysfunctional consultations

Consultation time (mins)	Phase II (mins)	Phase IV (mins)	Phase II (props)	Phase IV (props)
3·66	0·41	0	0·11	0
3·91	0·66	0·14	0·16	0·03
4·33	0·58	0·25	0·13	0·05
2·41	1·30	0	0·53	0
3·83	0·25	0	0·06	0
6·16	0·25	1·30	0·04	0·21
6·41	0·73	1·10	0·11	0·17
1·91	0·26	0	0·13	0
6·33	0·36	0·25	0·05	0·03
1·55	0·30	0	0·19	0
2·41	0·32	0	0·13	0
5·41	0·75	0·35	0·13	0·06
6·30	1·91	0·25	0·30	0·03
4·06	2·03	0·11	0·50	0·02
11·80	6·30	1·25	0·53	0·10
4·68	1·20	0·25	0·25	0·05
2·95	0·31	0·09	0·10	0·03
1·91	0·25	0	0·13	0
6·33	1·55	0·15	0·24	0·02
5·28	2·16	0·38	0·40	0·07
6·18	3·00	0	0·48	0
2·21	0·55	0·05	0·24	0·02
6·33	1·91	0·25	0·30	0·03
5·41	1·73	0	0·32	0
7·00	4·13	0	0·59	0
4·86	1·30	0·25	0·26	0·05
6·55	1·26	1·05	0·19	0·16
9·75	3·58	2·55	0·36	0·26
14·80	6·33	4·38	0·42	0·29
3·65	0·33	0·15	0·09	0·04
5·13	0·55	0·33	0·10	0·06
4·16	0·41	0·28	0·09	0·06
8·10	3·58	1·77	0·44	0·21
6·30	2·30	1·01	0·36	0·16
5·55	3·35	0·25	0·60	0·04
6·50	1·41	0·20	0·21	0·03
2·91	0·72	0	0·24	0
4·61	0·58	0·20	0·12	0·04
5·41	1·13	0·12	0·20	0·02

Dysfunctional consultations

Consultation time (mins)	Phase II (mins)	Phase IV (mins)	Phase II (props)	Phase IV (props)
3·30	0·20	0·25	0·06	0·07
2·10	0·34	0·38	0·16	0·18
3·59	1·11	0	0·43	0
3·05	0·09	0·09	0·03	0·03
4·10	0·10	0·15	0·02	0·03
6·30	1·60	0·25	0·25	0·04
3·10	1·35	0·15	0·44	0·05
3·25	1·10	0	0·34	0
4·30	1·10	0	0·26	0
3·10	0·25	0·36	0·08	0·11
3·03	0·33	0·52	0·10	0·17
4·07	0·09	0	0·02	0
3·70	0·42	0	0·11	0
2·50	0·26	0	0·06	0
2·57	0·20	0	0·07	0
3·35	0·28	0·35	0·08	0·10
3·25	0·10	0·38	0·03	0·11
3·39	0·30	0·35	0·08	0·10
3·65	0·16	0·92	0·04	0·25
2·25	0·50	0	0·22	0
4·25	1·19	0·36	0·28	0·11
6·25	0·30	1·25	0·04	0·02
2·55	0·12	0	0·04	0
6·07	0·70	0·95	0·11	0·15
4·02	0·10	0	0·02	0
4·45	0·42	0	0·09	0
3·85	1·12	0	0·29	0
4·59	1·37	0	0·30	0
4·80	0·13	1·20	0·02	0·25
5·60	0·50	0·85	0·08	0·15
5·00	0·39	0·75	0·07	0·15
4·20	0·33	0·80	0·07	0·19
8·20	1·85	3·25	0·22	0·39
6·10	0·60	0·63	0·09	0·10
4·90	0·15	0·25	0·03	0·05
6·25	2·40	0·40	0·38	0·06

CHAPTER 9

DOCTORS AND CONSULTING STYLES: GROUPING BEHAVIOURS (PART I)

So far we have concentrated our attention upon the overall design of the consultation and the individual items of behaviour which may go to make up that consultation. It is now necessary to examine the various ways in which the items of behaviour may be grouped.

Originally the intention was to reduce the list of behaviours identified to a manageable set of about twenty. This proved very difficult, because any reduction to this size reduced the sensitivity of the measuring instrument.

During this attempt at reduction another factor started to manifest itself which, in a totally different way, solved the problem of grouping. In order to explain this we need to look at three pairs of consultations. These consultations were provided by three different doctors, and the time gap between the first and second consultation is at least a week.

The first pair (Dr H——) are constructed around a very carefully organised pattern of questions. This doctor asks questions to clarify the problem which he thinks has been presented, and to eliminate various other problems which occur to him. What is significant is his inability to change his pattern of consulting even when confronted with a considerable flow of emotion during the interview.

(Each of the following consultations is written as it occurred in transcript from the audio-tape.)

Dr H——. *Example 1*

D. "Come in and sit down. What can we do for you?"

P. "It's not nerves, doctor. I'm sure it's not nerves. Last night. It was hurting me when I went to bed. I haven't been sick but I've had diarrhoea . . . it was just like water."

D. "Have you had the diarrhoea before?"

P. "I have, but not like this, this was just water. . . ."

D. "You don't usually get diarrhoea when you get to bed, do you?"

P. "No, I'm usually sick."

D. "Where do you get the pain, here?"

P. "Just here, yes. Well, it feels heavy. Just not right, you know."

D. "Is it worse on one side than the other? On the right side; does anything bring it on do you know?"

P. "No, not that I know of."

D. "You also get it on the other side, do you?"

P. "Yes, last night it seemed worse, just there, as though I've been kicked from the inside. I feel very hungry before I get the pain, I want to eat a lot. I don't feel hungry at all, and I've had nothing to eat. I've just no appetite, and it saps my energy."

D. "Any particular sort of foods upset you?"

P. "At one time I did knock off the fats; fatty foods, you know."

D. "Does it make any difference when you have them?"

P. "No, not really. Well, I put a bit of marg on and scrape it off again. . . ."

D. "Do you get any other trouble, apart from the pain and the sickness?"

75

P. "Well, I don't know whether this has anything to do with it. . . ." (Crying.) Telephone interruption.

D. "You were telling me you've had this discharge—how long have you had that?"

P. (Patient talking rapidly and indistinctly because she is still crying.) "I've had a D and C and I thought . . . and there it was . . . he said I should have told you. . . ."

At this point the patient is evidently trying to find the words, and perhaps courage, to say something which she has been repressing. The doctor sees what is happening and stops it firmly with a factual direct question which he refines into a nearly closed question.

D. "I see. Do you get any other stomach trouble? Do you get any indigestion, wind or any of that sort of stuff, belching, etc?"

P. "Well, I feel as if it is wind, well that's what sort of pain it is, or indigestion."

D. "Have you taken any indigestion medicine?"

P. "Yes, I have . . . well, I've been taking milk of magnesia most of the time."

D. "What effect did that have?"

P. "Well, the . . . feeling it doesn't get rid of it. Last night if I'd have taken it it would have come back before I got to sleep. Like last Saturday morning. It started at six o'clock and it didn't finish until two."

D. "Is it a continuous pain or coming and going?"

P. "No, all the time. About six to eight hours at a time."

D. "And what do you do when you get it?"

P. "Lie on the floor, pull my knees up to my chest until this part of my back touches the floor and rock."

D. "How do you feel when you haven't got the pain?"

P. "Smashing, well, it's gone." (Laughs.)

D. "All right. Just let me have a look at your tummy again. Take your clothes off. Do you have any trouble with your waterworks?"

P. "No. I just manage to get about three hours' sleep, get up and cope with two children and get breakfast ready. It's still tender here . . . examination. . . ."

Here she has introduced new information which is completely unrelated to anything she has said before and unrelated to any question of the doctor's. The doctor does not take any notice.

D. "I find it very difficult to put a label on this, you know. How do you feel about having an X-ray test, barium meal?"

The doctor has now made up his mind. He has decided to have an X-ray, and the fact that she had one two months prior to this interview is not going to shake him.

P. "I've had one."

D. "Oh, of course you have. I'd just forgotten."

P. "A couple of months ago."

D. "And that was all right wasn't it?"

P. "Yes."

D. "And what else can you do, do you know?"

P. "It's very painful, it really is."

D. "Well, all right, I think we'll arrange to have some further tests done . . . a card. . . . Take these tablets, I'd say take two every day whether you've got the pain or not, and I'll give you some quite strong ones to take, only at night, one, but don't take them unless you have to. All right?"

P. "Yes. I just can't sleep you know if I know I'm going to get it."

Again she has repeated something about her sleeping habits. The tablets he is prescribing are not sleeping tablets.

D. "Now keep on with those. If your tablets are done before you have your X-ray come and see me. If not, after you've had your X-ray, will you?"

P. "I'm sorry to always keep coming. . . . It's baffling me as well."

D. "Why do you keep saying sorry to cause you . . .?"

(Crying.) Confused noise. Someone called Margaret was mentioned.

D. "What do you think gives you that idea?"

P. "Well, I've done it myself, you know, crikey she's always here. . . ."

When this part of the consultation was replayed to the doctor he realised that the patient was not talking about herself but about her sister-in-law. That lady was seriously ill in hospital with a suspected stomach cancer. He failed to hear anything because he was intent upon concluding the interview. His next three questions are best described as "misc. prof. noises". He is writing another prescription and a reminder to himself to arrange X-rays.

D. "Why do you think you're always here?"

P. "Well, I've never been away recently. . . ."

D. "No, I mean the other people you used to know. . . ."

P. "Well . . . came in with a scratch on his arm and Margaret told him to use calamine and he came back thinking it was the miracle cure—I'm beginning to feel like him!"

D. "It doesn't seem to work on you though, does it? All right?"

He gets back into communication with the patient in the last few words.

P. "Right. When will the X-rays be?"

D. "They'll be in a week or so. Do you know what they will be?"

P. "Yes, it will be . . . kidneys. All right."

D. " 'Bye-bye."

In his next consultation we again see Dr H—— attempting to cope with a difficult patient problem, using his very mechanistic style. Every time this patient offers feeling or some sort of real insight into her problem he copes with a very direct factual question, even when they are clearly counter-productive.

Example 2

D. "Come in, good afternoon. Well, what can we do for you?"

P. "I just keep feeling sick all the time."

D. "How long have you felt like this?"

P. "Oh, it goes on and off. I have had it before."

D. "When did you start like this then?"

P. "I have been feeling rotten for a bit, this week-end."

D. "What do you call a bit? How long have you felt rotten?"

P. "It started the New Year off . . . and I have not got right since."

D. "You saw Doctor—— here in October; you were feeling sick then. Is that right?

P. "Yes."

D. "Is this the same sort of thing? How long before that did you first start feeling sick then? Was that the first time?"

77

P. "Yes."
D. "And have you had this on and off since then?"
P. "Yes."
D. "All right. Tell me all about it."
P. "I don't know what . . . I just feel sick and. . . ."
D. "Is this all day, in the mornings or . . .?"
    (Here he interrupts her just as she seems ready to start.)
P. "Well, it is more or less in the morning, and then it goes off, and then it
    comes back again. I feel that if I could be sick, I would be all right, but I
    can't be."
D. "Apart from feeling sick, how do you feel in yourself otherwise?"
    This is as near as Dr H—— can get to asking an open-ended question.
P. "A bit tired and irritable."
D. "Why do you think you feel like that?"
P. "I don't know."
    It seems now that his attempts to use open-ended techniques have failed and
he reverts to direct and closed questions.
D. "Do you sleep well?"
P. "Sometimes. Sometimes I can't sleep."
D. "Do you have trouble getting to sleep or waking up?"
P. "Well. . . ."
D. "If you feel tired or off, does that affect your tummy?"
P. "No, not really. If I can't sleep, I can't sleep."
D. "No, but does it make your tummy worse?"
P. "No."
D. "Why do you think you feel miserable?"
P. "I don't really know."
D. "Have you been worried about something?"
P. "No. I have nothing to worry about."
D. "How long have you been married?"
P. "Five months."
D. "And how are things going?"
P. "All right."
D. "Where are you living now?"
P. "13 . . . Street."
D. "And have you got your house sorted out?"
P. "No. Part of it needs remodernising. . . ."
D. "And are there any financial worries there?"
P. "No."
D. "Do you go out to work?"
P. "Yes."
    It now seems that he is having to guess at what may be causing her problem
by seeking out all the causes of anxiety he can cope with.
D. "And how have things been at work?"
P. "Well, not bad."
D. "And what was the trouble yesterday?"
P. "Oh, nothing really."
D. "Have your periods been all right, waterworks?"
P. "Yes."

D. "Apart from being sick at work, do you like your work?"
P. "Yes."
D. "What work do you do?"
P. "Filing clerk, and typing."
D. "How long have you worked . . .?"
P. "Six years."
D. ". . . your husband, is he quite well?"
P. "Yes."
D. "What are your views on having a family?"
P. "We want children."
D. "Do you? Do you use any form of family planning?"
P. "No."
D. "You are not on the pill?"
P. "No. We want them as soon as possible."
D. "Do you? Do you have any problems in your marriage?"

This is a classic example of a question which will produce a predictable answer. The sort of question he needs has to be phrased in such a way that a simple short answer is not possible.

P. "No."
D. "What do you think is causing this sickness?"
P. "I don't really know."
D. "How long have you known your husband?"
P. "Five years."
D. "Five years; you should know him by now. All right, can I have a look at your tummy. Hop up on the couch. How is your chest these days?"
P. "Well, I think I might be allergic to dogs."
D. "Why?"
P. "Well, when I am with dogs, I can't breathe."
D. "When do you go with dogs?"
P. "Well, my mother-in-law has a dog."
D. "I see."
P. "I only have to be in the house a few minutes and. . . ."
D. "It sounds like it. You are not allergic to your husband?"

Here he stepped in very quickly and asked a wholly irrelevant question about the husband. Mention of mother-in-law was a danger signal to be coped with in this fashion.

P. "No. Just dogs."
D. "Just hop on the couch, will you?"
    Confused noise.
D. "Do you tend to worry a lot?"
P. "Not really."
D. "What sort of a temperament do you think you have then?"
P. "I just get irritable for no reason."
D. "I am going to give you some tablets to be going on with. One, twice a day, and can take a third one, but basically it is one twice a day, for a couple of weeks, and then come back to see me. Do you need a note for your work?"
P. "Just a sick note."
D. "How long are you thinking of staying off your work?"
P. "I will go back Thursday. . . . Just to say what is wrong."

D. "What is wrong with you?"
P. "I don't know."
D. "Goodbye."

An inconclusive end to a very odd consultation. A study of this doctor and his consultation shows that every consultation is made up of the same sort of questions and any intrusion of feeling or risk of emotive content is rapidly countered by a closed question about some new issue. The patient has no room to manoeuvre at all because the doctor is defining exactly the limits of her behaviour.

The next pair of interviews are of a doctor (Dr U——) who, when on training programmes, is constantly criticised by his peers for his over-use of reassurances. His voice and indeed his mannerisms do appear to have a very soothing effect upon the patient. In addition to this he is also prone, on occasions, to administer large doses of verbal reassurance.

In these two interviews we are not concerned with his use of reassurance but with his style. Dr H—— proceeded rapidly through a well controlled catechism. Dr U—— does have a short period of catechising but then moves away from this in an attempt to get the patient to verbalise a little feeling. In his first consultation (Example 3), if we examine the starred extract we can see that he uses this approach to make the patient consider a long-term solution which is already in his mind. He does need some degree of skill to make the patient talk in order to discover how acceptable his solution is. What also needs to be noted is the fact that even though he is making the patient talk he is still very much in control.

Dr U——. *Example 3*

D. "Come in. Hello dear. Now how are we doing?"
P. "Oh, well, I just feel the same really, doctor. I finished my period on the Tuesday and I should have started my period again on the Sunday normally, if I had have taken the pill for a complete month I should have started last Sunday, and I did, for four days. You know, the last time I came to see you you said we would probably have a clear month while I've finished taking this Gyna . . . but I should have started again with another period on the Sunday, which I did. But I've been okay since from Sunday until Wednesday."
D. "From Sunday until Wednesday. Now, let's be clear. I saw you three weeks ago and then your period lasted four days and you had; when did you start to bleed then?"
P. "On the Sunday. I came to see you on the Friday. I'd been on the sick for a week and you signed me off on the Friday."
D. "Yes, and you started on the Sunday and that carried on for what, four days?"
P. "Four days."
D. "And you started the pill on Wednesday, didn't you?"
P. "Yes."
D. "You've had no bleeding since that Sunday then? That's the eleventh of March."
P. "No."

80

D. "Right, then you're about three-quarters way through your packet at the moment?"

P. "Yes. I think I finish taking the packet one day next week. I think it's next Wednesday or Thursday, I'm not quite sure. I know it's one day next week."

D. "Well, I think things will work out all right. I think so. Come and see me again in about three weeks, will you, and let me know how your periods are going, but looks as if we might have altered this for you."

P. "Yes."

*D. "How many children have you got?"

P. "One."

D. "Just the one. Do you want any more?"

P. "Well, I do. I'm a bit like that whether I want to come off the pill or not, but you see I'm working just at the moment and we're saving up for things that we need. You know, but I would like another one now, you know, but I'm a bit like this at the moment, you know I would come off the pill."

D. "Well look, we're having a lot of trouble with the pill, haven't we really with this breakthrough. If you feel like that why not get your other baby over with and then you probably feel that two is all you want."

P. "Yes."

D. "You don't want any more?"

*P. "No."

D. "Well, my advice to you is—don't stop the pill now, I mean wait until the end of the packet, but if you really feel like that I would advise you to stop the pill, have your family and after you've had your baby be sterilised. You've got your family."

P. "You know, we'll have to talk this over."

D. "That seems sensible."

P. "You know, we've talked about this sterilisation and I feel I would like to be sterilised after I've had another child."

D. "Well, let's do it, while you're young enough."

P. "Yes."

D. "Okay. So come and see me when you start the period. Come and see me in your week's rest. Let me know how you're going on. We'll discuss then stopping the pill, going ahead trying to achieve a family, achieve a baby, and then, if you like, we'll sterilise you. And I think you'll be a lot happier."

P. "Oh, I think so, yes, it's making me feel a bit upside down, you know, with keep having a break, and then you know having the bleeding for four days, and being okay and then I don't. . . ."

D. "I think we'll stop it, you know. I think we will. We'll make a final decision in a fortnight."

P. " 'Bye, thanks very much doctor."

D. " 'Bye love."

In the next consultation we see Dr U——— performing in a very similar manner. He relies very heavily upon an apparent collaboration with his patient which becomes more evident after he has used his skill in getting his patient to talk. Apart from his greeting he does not use "we" until he is clear about his intended course of action. He requires her collaboration in so far as he expects her to agree with his prognosis.

Example 4

D. "Come in. Now then, how are we doing?"

P. "Just the same really."

D. "You're obviously no better, are you? How are things progressing?"

P. "Not so bad."

D. "What about the bungalow?"

P. "Coming along all right."

D. "Is it taking shape? When do you think you'll be able to be in?"

P. "In the next month, I hope. There's such a lot to do before we can go in."

D. "That's not too bad. Do you mean the beginning of April?"

P. "Well, I hope so anyway."

D. "Well, your problems aren't really going to alter, are they, until you get into your bungalow. How are the relationships with your mother now, are they still . . .?"

P. "Just the same, although I am not as bothered."

D. "How does she react to your going into a home of your own?"

P. "She's a bit bothered that I won't be able to cope. She keeps putting me off the idea. I'll have to look after myself and the baby and don't let myself slip back."

D. "Is she putting you off?"

P. "She is in a way, really."

D. "She is in a way. You don't feel very confident do you?"

P. "No, not at the moment."

D. "Do you think that M—— will give you any help?"

P. "He'll have to, really."

D. "Do you think he will continue on as a musician, or will he take a job?"

P. "I'm hoping he will take a job. I've mentioned it to him but he just wants to keep on being a musician. Nothing I say can change his mind."

D. "Well, it's not a bad job provided he has a regular job. At the moment it doesn't seem to be regular, does it?"

P. "Not really."

D. "So why not let. . . . Don't you think it might be a good thing if he carried on being a musician, but a regular musician?"

P. "There are so many problems that bother me really. I want to get out myself, really, and get some extra money."

D. "You have so many problems haven't you?"

P. "I suppose I make more of them than I should do."

D. "Well, these problems are present in everybody's life, and you know, once you move into this bungalow a lot of these are going to disappear of themselves."

Pause.

D. "Have you got enough tablets?"

Dr U—— has now made up his mind and is starting to enter into his "collaborative phase".

P. "I've got enough."

D. "You've got enough. Okay. Can you manage over for a fortnight's time?"

P. "Yes."

D. "And we hope by then with a bit of luck you may be in your house by then."

82

P. "Mmm, maybe."

D. "Then we can really start, can't we?"

P. "Yes."

D. "Do you think you feel any better now?"

P. "Well, some days I do and some days I don't. I don't know. I think a lot and my mind starts wondering over all sorts of things. That's why I think I'll be better when I'm in the cottage because I'll have more to do and more to occupy my mind. I have a lot of spare time on my hands and when baby's asleep I start getting depressed and start worrying."

D. "Don't worry. Give it another fortnight and I'll see you again. Bring M—— with you next time, will you? I'd like to see him, it's some time since I've seen him. So will you bring him next time? 'Bye love"

The third pair of example consultations were provided by a doctor who utilises a very rare style indeed. His style is odd but so is his insistence upon not running a surgery with any sort of rigid appointment system or even a notional system of time allocation. Patients come on a day rather than at a time. He belongs to a group of not more than 1 per cent of our sample which has an average patient consultation time in excess of 10 minutes.

In this set of examples we will observe a very extensive pattern of questions designed to clarify the reason for the patient being there. Slowly as the doctor progresses into Phase III the nature of his questioning changes and he starts to use suggestion and lots of encouraging noise.

In Example 5 it will also be noted that this patient is not the most communicative person to enter a surgery. It is probably true to say that he would prefer a doctor with a much more closed style like Dr H——. Despite this, the doctor presses on with his approach, continually forcing the patient to talk.

This approach changes very suddenly once the doctor has made up his mind about the patient because he starts to present the patient with a very complex mixture of information and opinion concerning his problems.

Dr C——. *Example 5*

Six seconds of confused noise.

D. "Come in. Do sit down. It's Mr (two seconds confused noise) Mr Be?"

P. "No. Mr Ba."

D. "Here I am. That's right. Now do sit down. There's two medical students.'

P. "Yeah."

D. "What can I do for you?"

P. "I had a cold which went to my head. . . ."

D. "Mmm."

P. "Six weeks ago. I'm aiming to get rid of it."

D. "Mmm."

P. "Feverish head pains."

D. "When was the fever and the pain?"

P. "I have been having them during the day."

D. "For how long, six weeks?"

P. "No. No, it's been getting worse recently."

D. "Mmm."

P. "About the last five days."

D. "You bring phlegm up when you cough?"

P. "No. No, I haven't been coughing."

D. "You haven't been coughing? You've been hot?"

P. "No."

D. "Short of breath?"

P. "Never noticed."

D. "You said it was not in your chest."

P. "No."

D. "What particular chest symptoms have you?"

P. (Pause.) "I'm not sure I know what you mean."

D. "Well, you (next few words inaudible), you remember that you said that you don't have a cough and you're not short of breath."

P. "Oh, oh, I see. No, but I had a cold and a cough."

D. "Yes."

P. "And I felt pain further down."

D. "Yes."

P. "And so on. The cold's gone (next few words inaudible) but I still have this."

D. "Yes. You still have the pain."

P. "Yes."

D. "It's just pains in your chest as far as your chest is concerned."

P. "Yeah."

D. "Which part of your chest?"

P. "Oh, mostly up here."

D. "So it's up there that we go to work." (Next few words inaudible.)

P. "No, it isn't. It's here."

D. "Just further, and it depends on the time?"

P. "No."

D. "Can you tell me where about?"

P. "Mmm." (Pause.) "I get, felt tight. Tight feeling."

D. "Mmm."

P. "And sort of burning tight."

D. "Mmm."

P. "Throughout. Back of the throat and down."

D. "Mmm."

P. "And then feverish."

D. "At the same time as the pain you felt feverish?"

P. "Yeah."

D. "And then do the two go away together as well?"

P. "Yes."

D. "And the pain lasts for how long, you know, about five minutes or a whole day?"

P. "Five minutes."

D. "For about five minutes. Can you think of any reason why it should be happening, you know, is there anything on your mind about it?"

P. "No. I thought I had an infection or something."

D. "Ah, is it any different when you're standing up or lying down?"

P. "No."

D. "Does anything make any difference to it, that is, make it better or worse?"

P. "No."

D. "No. Anything, is there anything that can precipitate an attack of the tightness and burning?"
P. "No."
D. "No. Okay. And when you've got it there's nothing can make it any better? You just have to wait for it to go?"
P. "Mmm."
D. "What do you do when it's there?"
P. "I worry."
   Patient laughs a little.
D. "You worry?"
P. "Yeah."
D. "Does it stop you doing what you were doing before?"
P. "No."
D. "You can carry on doing what you were doing. Is it likely to occur when you're out doing something during the day or when you're sitting down doing nothing?"
P. "I haven't noticed. I. . . ." (Next few words inaudible.)
D. "Oh, yes. When you worry, what do you worry about?"
P. "Oh, about my chest."
D. "Mmm."
P.   (Few words inaudible.)
D. "Yeah. And what about the chest pains, do you worry?"
P. "Oh, well, I really don't know."
D. "Nothing specific like?"
P. "No."
D. "Worrying it's TB or worrying it's a growth, or that kind of thing?"
P. "No. No, I don't have any of those problems."
D. "You have other problems?"
*P. (Short laugh.) "I won't say in here."
D. "Do you think they might be (words inaudible)?"
*P. (Short laugh, then both laughing.)
   The starred sequence is quite an interesting approach to the problem of relieving the tremendous tension the doctor has managed to build up. He allows the patient to make his little joke and then capitalises, so that both are laughing. That part of the consultation is then over.
D. "Okay, let's have a look at your chest."
   Two minutes of confused noise whilst a physical examination takes place.
   Note now how his style changes completely.
D. "Right. Well. Ah, assessment at the moment of the pains is that they don't reflect any chest disease at all. I can't hear anything wrong, they don't sound from the way you talk about them as typical of any kind of chest illness and I would like to confirm that by X-raying your chest and I think that will. I'm expecting the X-ray to be clear and I think that would dispose of any idea of any trouble in your chest."
P. "Mmm."
D. "It may be that you aren't right when you say that your problems aren't relevant to this, one of them could be because obviously if you've got symptoms we've got to account for them and if there's no physical illness there to account for them there must be some other reason."

85

P. "Mmm."

D. "Ah, could we get this X-ray out of the way, and assume that, have you back and if it's negative as I'm guessing it will be, will we take if from there, eh? Okay?"

P. "Yes."

D. "If you have an X-ray done now it will be a few days before I get the report through, but you can have it done while you're here this morning. (Pause for one minute, doctor writing.) You know the staircase where you came in, the staircase near the waiting-room where you were, if you go up there on the first floor you will see a big notice saying X-ray."

P. "Mmm."

D. "Okay. If you'd like to go and hand that to them they will take a picture and I will have the report in, say, about five days' time or something like that, and if you could come back then I will let you have the report on the X-ray and we can see how things are doing and do anything further that seems necessary."

P. "Fine."

D. "Okay. That's it. Now come back on . . . let me see, today's Thursday, any time from next Tuesday on. Okay?"

P. "Thank you."

Example consultation 6 from Dr C—— is an example of how he copes with repeat prescriptions. He already has detailed information on this patient, but as we shall see he also has a few reservations, particularly about what to prescribe. Note again how he quickly and easily gets this patient to talk but also how he keeps his purpose in mind by forcing the patient to answer a question which seemed to have been avoided.

Example 6

D. "Come in."

P. "It's a Dr . . . ?"

D. "Yes. Come in Mr F——. Do sit down. These are two different medical students from the two you met last time."

P. "Oh, you have cooled me down a lot, a lot better. Now I can concentrate better and everything. The nervous system, everything is going fine."

D. "That's nice. No trouble at all. Any flies in the ointment at all?"

P. No, nothing. I'll probably be all right. The tablets suit me down to the ground until I really get used to them. That's the only trouble I think. I'm taking two a day as you said."

D. "Yes."

P. "All I get is a bit of a taste in my mouth."

D. "Mmm."

P. "I take a drop of orange juice or something like that."

D. "When you say you're frightened you get used to them, is that. . . ?"

P. "Will I keep being as active as I am now at the moment? I'm very active like. I can concentrate better, my nervous system is a lot better."

D. "Mmm."

P. "And I can think clear, more clearly. I'm not worried like I was before, you see what I mean, more settled."

D. "Mmm."

86

P. "Since I've been taking these tablets."

D. "Yes."

P. "The others that I was taking as you said weren't any good. It was just for the nervous system, the tension you see."

D. "Mmm."

P. "And I still get them sinking feeling pains in my stomach you see."

D. "Is there a feeling 'this is too good to be true'?"

P. "No, well I think it's, they're very good. I'd say they're very good. The only effect is this fish taste like. I take them three or four hours after." (Few words inaudible.)

D. "Mmm."

P. "You know, but I take like a drop of tea or a drink of orange juice."

D. "So?"

P. "Or something like that."

D. "No, I was pursuing that remark you made about you might get too used to them."

P. "Aye."

D. "Is that based on the kind of feeling 'it can't last'?"

P. "No. No. But you can get used to a drug you see what I mean, you can get used to them like they'd have no effect, you'd have to take more and more that's what I mean."

D. "Mmm."

P. "You see, to do the same work."

D. "Mmm. Has that happened to you in the past?"

P. "No. No. No."

D. "Is it something you've heard about from other people?"

P. "Well, I imagine so. Now common sense would tell me so."

D. "Mmm."

P. "But what as they are now two a day are doing me very well."

D. "You take two together?"

P. "No. I take one. One in the morning."

D. "One in the morning and one at night?"

P. "Yes. Oh, I don't take two of them all together because I realise they're pretty strong."

D. "Mmm. It would be okay actually to take the two together at night, and in fact what I can do, since you've nearly finished those, is to give you some of the double strength ones so that you don't even have to take those, you can take one at night of the double strength ones."

P. "Oh, I see. Right."

D. "Be just as good."

P. "Well, I've got six left, so I won't want. . . ."

D. "Yeah."

P. "I only want about twenty, nineteen, won't I? You allowed me twenty-five last time."

D. "Yeah. I can give you some more this time."

P. "Right oh."

D. "The first time I gave you them I was, I didn't give you all that many because it was just the possibility you might have decided to take them all at once."

87

P. "No."
D. "No."
P. "I wouldn't do that."
D. "Well, you know, I didn't know you then at all. It was a thought in my mind."
P. "I've had my lesson. Saw it. When I was inside there where I had my shock treatment I seen some of them poor wretches in there. Brought me to my heel right away, you see I realised then how sorry I was. It's very important."
(Fifteen seconds have been deleted whilst the doctor checks on patient's address with his receptionist.)
D. "Yeah. Okay. These are the same thing but they're double strength, and they're just like two of the others rolled into one."
P. "That's fine, thank you. So I'll just take one."
D. "Just take one."
P. (Words inaudible.)
D. (Words inaudible.) ". . . and could I see you in a fortnight?"
P. "A fortnight, yeah. Thank you, doctor. Thank you very much indeed Good morning all."
D. "Okay, good morning."

What stands out in these three pairs of consultations is the degree to which any given consultation conducted by a particular doctor is like another consultation conducted by the same doctor.

What follows are three extracts from consultations provided by each of these three doctors. They were extracted at random from a collection of transcripts. Identifying which doctor is which is not difficult.

Extract 1

P. "Well then, I felt that I ought to go and see her again."
D. "Mmm."
P. "When I did I felt the same as before."
D. "Mmm. Go on."
P. "Well she was like she used to be. Too much make-up—you know. So I spoke to her."
D. "Yes?"

Extract 2

D. "How do you feel about stopping smoking?"
P. "Well, I've really cut it down, you know."
D. "Now's your chance. Have you finished the capsules Doctor X gave you?"
P. "Well, I'm down to my last one."
D. "And are you taking those little pink ones?"
P. "The little pink ones, yes."
D. "How many are you taking a day of those?"
P. "Three of those."
D. "Yes. Have you got some of those left?"
P. "Oh. Yes."

Extract 3

D. "You came last time and you told me, how much were you overdue . . . ?"
P. "I was three weeks last time and I'm five weeks over now."
D. "You're five over. So your last period was. . . ."
P. "About the eighteenth of January."

88

D. "Now let me see, the last time you came you didn't just tell me about it."
P. "No, I kept being sick."
D. "You were being sick, weren't you?"
P. "I still keep being. . . ."
D. "And I gave you some tablets, didn't I?"

Identifying the doctors is clearly not difficult. All we are doing is recognising the way in which a person has learned to talk to another person and the degree to which it has a measure of predictability. It is the repetitive quality and the predictability which constitutes a style.

The question must then be asked, "What is a style?" Most of the doctors we have studied have been in practice for at least 10 years. None of them received any particular training in the art of consulting and thus learned to consult patients the "hard way". The consultation is a repetitive activity. It would seem reasonable to suggest that after a period of time doctors learn a package of behaviours which seem to work in most instances and this package then appears to become ossified.

This very much accords with what we would expect of anyone learning a repetitive activity, but as we can see in example consultation No 1 there are severe strains when the style is inappropriate to the problem. While the patient here is in an emotional state and is clearly ready to talk, the doctor does not have the range of behaviour to exploit the situation. Equally in example consultation No 5 the patient is not a great talker and the doctor might well consider whether his effort was worth the result. The way in which a doctor sets about a consultation is, however, largely repetitive. Certainly, as we have already noted, his greeting is idiosyncratic and also repetitive, as is the rest of his consultation, but in a different way.

Let us return to our six consultations and look at the way in which each doctor asks questions. Doctor H—— uses a lot of direct and closed questions. He occasionally ventures an open question or a search for a patient's idea but rarely follows up or pursues the answer. Take, for example, one such effort in example consultation No 2:

D. "Apart from feeling sick, how do you feel in yourself otherwise?"
P. "A bit tired and irritable."
D. "Why do you feel like that?"
P. "I don't know."
D. "Do you sleep well?"

In this extract the doctor has tried a fairly open-ended approach but his second attempt produced very little. Consequently, instead of increasing the pressure by another open-ended question or even a silence he is back into his normal mode with a closed question. "Do you sleep well?" is a shot in the dark which produces nothing.

Dr U—— is quite different. He does, of course, ask his questions, but he then starts to use a suggestive technique to get the patient to produce answers he probably wants but will not impose.

For example: "Well, let's do it while you're young enough."

Dr C——, however, is an open-ended questioner and an encouraging mumbler. His concern is to get the patient to talk and talk until sufficient information has been generated to allow the doctor to decide what should happen next.

The three doctors provided nearly fifty consultations each. It would be quite wrong to claim that every consultation was identical, but it is possible to claim that the majority of consultations they submitted are constructed in a similar fashion.

Another phenomenon which is repeated centres upon that point in the consultation at which the doctor finally makes his own private decisions about the patient. This decision might be a diagnosis, or it may be a decision to refer the patient to some other agency or it may simply be a recognition of the fact that he is not going to make a diagnosis.

If we refer back to our examples once more it is possible to identify the point at which these doctors make their decisions. Once they have done their private decision-making, they drop the style they are using and adopt a new style. Let us compare Dr H—— with Dr C——. Dr H—— pursues a series of questions until he makes a decision. He then terminates the consultation fairly quickly. Dr C—— is quite different. He spends a lot of his time making the patient talk and simply listening. When he makes his mind up he will then start to talk at some length.

If a consultation is proceeding through its six phases (see Chapter 3) the point at which the doctor would make his decision would coincide approximately with the termination of the verbal and physical examination, ie Phase III. The style a doctor uses to make his diagnosis is not necessarily the style he uses to prescribe. Dr James MacCormick (now Professor of Community Medicine at Trinity College, Dublin) once attended a complete course on counselling and commented afterwards that he used the counselling technique solely to improve his diagnosis. He was not in the least enamoured of counselling as a prescribing process. That, he said "was the doctor's job". As we shall see, this is not an uncommon view.

In order to study the way in which doctors group their units of behaviour into patterns we must now start to look at the consultation in two parts. Initially we are going to look at that part of a consultation prior to the doctor making his decisions.

Phases I, II and III

These phases (relating to the patient; discovering reasons for attendance; physical and verbal examination) are part of the process the doctor uses to ensure that he knows what decisions to make about the patient condition. It is possible to identify a range of styles which can be said to typify the management of these stages. These styles are not watertight compartments. However, as a spectrum of styles it is noticeable that doctors operate in preferred segments of that spectrum.

If we think about any consultation there are normally two parties—the doctor and the patient. The doctor has special skills and experience which may well be the key component of that consultation. It is wise to remember that the patient too has a unique pattern of knowledge and experience and any consultation is made up of a mixture of the patient and the doctor. The relationship between the two may be described by the following diagram:

90

Figure 1

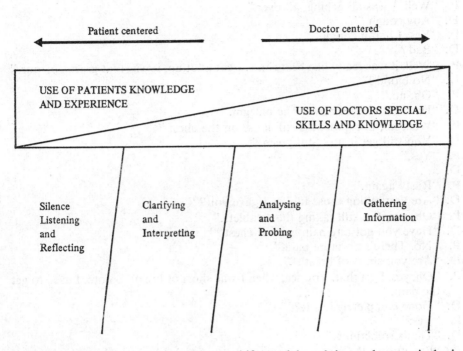

This model is known as a power-shift model and is used extensively in sociology and organisation psychology.

(The titles given to the four basic styles of diagnostic behaviour should not be confused with the individual behaviours as presented earlier.)

The four basic styles are essential, ideal models which are never quite the same in practice. For example, a doctor who uses a "gathering information" style will have a number of analytic and probing patterns of behaviour as well possibly, as a little clarifying. These other styles, however, will be very secondary and will not constitute a substantial part of his "normal" behaviour (*vide* Dr H——).

Let us look at some example consultations which illustrate these various styles and also illustrate the degree to which a particular style is not absolutely watertight. Let us look firstly at a doctor who normally spends his time *gathering information*. In this case the complete consultation is offered because the ending is extremely significant.

Dr R——.

D. "Come in, please, come in and sit down. No better?"

P. "I don't know what was the matter, but I've had a fortnight in bed."

D. "With what?"

P. "With 'flu."

D. "'Flu?"

P. "I lost my balance."

D. "And how did this 'flu affect you?"

91

P. "I was sweating and sneezing, I couldn't stop sneezing."

D. "Any aches and pains?"

P. "Well, I was all aching, all over."

D. "Any cough?"

P. "Yes, I had a cough."

D. "Bad?"

P. "Well, it was really like bronchitis. I got a lot up, it was that greeny colour."

D. "No blood?"

P. "Oh, no."

D. "Has that cleared now? The phlegm."

P. "Well, no, not quite, it's still loose on the chest."

D. "You still get it up? Still green?"

P. "Yes."

D. . . . .

P. "Rusty again."

D. "Are you taking those tablets I gave you?"

P. "Oh, yes, I'm still taking those tablets."

D. "Have you got any pain in your chest?"

P. "No. There's no more pain."

D. "Are you short of breath?"

P. "Oh, yes, I get that. You see, when I was short of breath before, I used to get the pain."

D. "Gone completely has it?"

P. "Yes."

D. "That's something."

P. "But during the night, sometimes, I can feel it like catarrh at the back of my throat. But that looks brown."

D. "Does it wake you? Your chest?"

P. "Well, it's not this last few nights."

D. "These little white tablets, have you any left?"

P. "No. . . ."

D. "What's your weight doing now, steady?"

P. "Well, as a matter of fact, doctor, we were weighing ourselves last night, my husband and I, and he said, 'What weight are you,' and I said, 'According to those I'm only eight stone,' and we put it past the zero and it was only eight stone odd."

D. . . . .

P. "So I don't think . . . the scale for a while. I think I was eight stone two when you weighed me last."

D. "You are eight stone four, you have lost a bit."

P. "Yes, I have."

At this point the doctor has made up his mind and is about to move into a prescriptive phase. He has a clear strategy in his mind and now becomes very insensitive to the various offers (starred) made by the patient.

D. "That's reasonable, because the thyroid tablets. . . . I'll make a note of that. Well, keep on the white tablets, one a day. I'll give you some tablets and medicine to clear your chest, the instructions will be on the bottle."

P. ". . . everyone has a cold."

D. "It's a bad time of year; you take the tablets four times a day and the medicine according to the instructions, I think you'll find that will clear it. There is enough there anyway for about a week. If you are not 100 per cent certain you must come back. But the little white tablets you must take permanently. So see how you get on and if you're not happy come back in a week."

*P. "I see Andrew's had a bad cold, hasn't he?"

D. "Has he?"

*P. "He's still sniffly."

D. "Well, it's the time of year for it, you can't expect. . . ."

P. ". . . but I could have done with trying those 'flu injections. . . ."

D. "It's too late this year now."

P. "Yes, it's too late."

D. "About November."

P. "I'll come in then."

D. "Well, last year was a good year for 'flu and this year isn't so good."

*P. "My throat is a bit. . . ."

D. "When you get an infection you will always get this rustiness. . . ."

*P. "I noticed that. . . . Dr—— told me I had a relaxed throat. I had to not speak as much and stop singing so I can't get the high notes now. All my notes have gone."

D. " 'Bye now."

In this interview it is very difficult for the patient to offer much more than answers to the rather closed questions from the doctor. This doctor in all of his consultations demonstrates this style and is prepared to deny the value of any greater patient involvement. A discussion with this doctor, who is incidentally a GP trainer, produced the following statement:

"The doctor's primary task is to manage his time. If he allows patients to rabbit on about their conditions then the doctor will lose control of time and will spend all his time sitting in a surgery listening to irrelevant rubbish. Effective doctoring is characterised by a 'quick clean job'."

In a morning surgery this doctor will see patients at a rate in excess of one every five minutes. His appointment system schedules up to 14 per hour and, he claims, people rarely have to wait long.

This style is extremely dependent upon the skill of the doctor in deciding very early on the reason for the patient being there. The next example, by the same doctor as the last, is included as an illustration of how dangerous this style can be. This is a fascinating consultation with an old man of about 70 who has been on this doctor's list since he took the practice over many years previously. There is, therefore, a long relationship. The patient had not made an appointment and should have attended for a regular check two weeks later. All through the consultation the doctor assumes that the patient is there simply to pick up his regular prescription.

D. "Hello, come in, how are you?"

P. "Got a cold. . . ."

D. "It's the fashion this week, everybody's got it. Well, now, how's the breathing going, any different?"

P. "Not so bad, doctor, can't grumble, I feel a bit better than I did before."

D. "That's a good sign. Are you coughing at all?"

93

P. "A bit. Just got a bad chest, just my arms you know."

D. "It's the cold and damp—that sort of thing. You didn't have an appointment did you?"

P. "Oh, on Friday I had a letter from them saying that they've altered my appointment—they've altered it and brought it forward. . . ."

D. "They've brought it from the fifteenth of March to the thirteenth of March—that's a funny postponement isn't it, unless they've reorganised the clinic—Dr Walker's away, anyway—probably a misprint . . . are you taking those tablets, one in a morning, one heart tablet, three of . . . two of the other one and a spoonful of medicine, yes, well I would like you to carry on with those unless Doctor Walker wants you to change. Well, that's the fifteenth. I'll see you again before you go to the out-patients there and we'll see how things are going."

P. "Will you see me before . . .?"

D. "Well, you're going on the thirteenth. That's the same day, isn't it, that's also on Tuesday four weeks today. Well, if you make an appointment for, say, the Thursday, the fifteenth, tell me what he has to say, that will be better . . . he didn't mention in his letter but very often he just forgets and lets the secretary sort it out. 'Bye-bye."

Again this case has been discussed at length with the doctor concerned and with a group of five other doctors. It was the cause of considerable discussion and criticism by the group. The major criticism was that the doctor never once attempted to use any reflecting behaviour or seek patient ideas. He also appears to use his reassurance in order to "close off" every single offer made by the patient. He also appears to assume that he understands the exact nature of the patient problem and uses reassurance to justify his own assumptions.

The offer of "a cold" by the patient can reasonably be seen as an opening overture in order to establish a legitimate cause for attending the surgery. The response from the doctor can be viewed as a straight dismissal of the importance of such a symptom. Next the doctor asks a question related to a previous examination. The patient responds with some information, which is met with some reassurance and a supplementary question from the doctor.

The patient's reply to the question about coughing produces two pieces of information which caused a great dispute in the peer group. "The chest" could be regarded as information related to the question, but the peer group argued "the arms" were not. Once again it will be observed the doctor uses "reassurance" to stop any further development.

So far, what seems to be happening is that the patient is trying to tell the doctor that he has some totally new symptoms but the doctor is not inclined to accept these and is still pursuing another line of enquiry.

The next interaction is much more significant. The question about the appointment is provoked by the doctor reading his case notes and recognising that the patient was there two weeks early. The patient, however, grasps this opportunity to express some of his anxiety about an out-patient appointment which had been changed.

The doctor accurately diagnosed a little anxiety in the patient but his method of managing that anxiety is very strange, if only because his first attempt can only heighten that anxiety. Recognising his error he then tries to cover up with an excuse. Then he very quickly switches to treatment and tries to close the interview. The patient is not prepared to close. The doctor, instead of dealing with the issue he has largely created, defers for a month.

During the discussion of this case the doctor claimed that what he learned from the interview was his need to utilise a clarifying strategy. He then proceeded to defend the consultation by pointing out that he was running beyond his allocated time and that the deferment was used in order to allow the patient a full five minutes at the next interview.

The majority of the doctors we have studied use the "information gathering" style or the "analysing and probing" style we are to examine now. In very few cases do we find a clear-cut and pure example of either style. More commonly we find doctors moving backwards and forwards between the two. In the next extract we will examine a doctor pursuing a completely non-medical line of questioning mainly in an analysing and probing style. The difference between this style and the previous style may be seen in the way in which each of the questions asked by the doctor is a development upon the previous question. Another interesting feature is the patient offering up a "desirable medical symptom" before actually letting the doctor know why she is really there.

D. "Come in. What can I do for you?"

P. "Well, I have got 'flu, doctor. I have got all pains in my arms."

D. "When did you start to feel not so well?"

P. "The week-end. It started Saturday afternoon, shivering with cold. . . . I came mostly about my head, it is paining me a lot. My husband . . . with a shoe, it cut me there, I couldn't comb my hair or touch my hair."

D. "Oh, dear, when was this?"

P. "Saturday night."

D. "How come?"

P. "He came home drunk as usual. He has hit me in the past, but not for a long while . . . causing trouble . . . people next door banging on the walls and it is getting on my nerves."

D. "Does he drink much during the week?"

P. "Not so much during the week, but at week-ends. Saturday and Sunday."

D. "Does he drink beer or spirits?"

P. ". . . It is a young couple next door . . . disturbing them . . . banging on the walls and this is affecting my nerves."

D. "Does he drink at all during the week?"

P. "Well, maybe once or twice."

D. "Does he get drunk then?"

P. "Not bad."

This example of probing was recorded by a doctor who can easily use a reflecting technique. (The example we offer later of reflecting was recorded by this doctor.) Occasionally he does "slip-up" (his own description) and stand on his dignity. In the next example we see the effect of not discovering why the patient was there. The patient is a young boy of 10 or 11 who has turned up in the surgery without a parent. The doctor could find nothing wrong with the child and was prescribing a near-useless bottle of cough mixture when the real reason was offered. (See *—*.)

D. "Come in. Hello. Take a seat. What can we do for you?"

P. "Well, I have got a cough, and I don't feel like eating with it."

D. "Have you got a cold in your nose? No. Can you take your coat off for me, and I'll just have a listen. How long have you had your cough?"

P. "Two weeks."

D. "How do you like the snow. No?"

P. "No."

D. "Too cold?"

P. "Yes."

D. "A big breath, good, again. Now round the back. Thanks very much. All right, I will give you some medicine to go on four times a day, will you?"

P. "... X-rays."

D. "X-rays, why X-rays?"

P. "My mum said. . . ."

D. "Your mum said. Why, was she worried?"

P. "Yes."

D. "Why, what did she say was the matter?"

P. "Well, I don't. . . ."

D. "Does anyone in your family have any chest trouble?"

P. "No."

D. "Well, tell your mum, you have this medicine for a week and then to come back and see me. If you are no better then, we will get your chest X-rayed. But I think it will cure with the medicine, because the X-rays won't make you better will they?"

P. "No."

D. "Tell the lady at the desk you have got to come back in a week. All right? 'Bye."

The doctor was very irritated that the child had been sent alone when the real patient was the mother. During the discussion of this case the doctor felt that had he probed just a little more when his physical examination produced nothing he might have found out a little earlier why the child was there.

We have also to consider one further concept here, and that is the needs of the patient. Some sort of "felt needs" must cause the patient to visit the doctor and part of any consultation ought to be the problem of finding out what these needs might be.

One may illustrate this point by reference to two transcripts above. In the first example we observed the doctor not acting upon the first statement made by the patient, but choosing to pursue a probing and clarifying strategy. This approach very quickly generated the information concerning the real reasons for attendance—which had nothing to do with influenza.

In his second interview, because he was pressed for time, he was well into his physical examination before the real causes for the patient's attendance were made clear.

Clarifying and interpreting strategies are much more rare than anything we have examined to date. Over 75 per cent of the doctors studied in this project use a style which is based upon the two previous styles. Of the remaining 25 per cent, only one in five is capable of a true reflecting style. The most common approach to a patient-centred style is the style we are about to examine. Occasional acts of "clarifying and interpreting" do occur in consultations which are very doctor-centred. In only a few consultations, however, is the style consistent throughout the whole consultation.

The following example is taken from a very complicated and difficult consultation. The whole consultation can be interpreted as an attempt to enable the patient to clarify the root causes of her own problems.

D. "Well, Mrs T——."

P. "I don't know really where to start to tell you. I have pains in my stomach, that's nothing very much. But on Monday I would have tried to commit suicide if I could have managed it."

D. "Why was that? Why did you feel so bad?"

P. "I am sorry." (Crying.)

D. "That's quite all right."

P. "I know it is very stupid and foolish. . . . I haven't been sleeping well for some months, I get very tired during the day and yet when I go to bed I don't sleep. It is kind of, you know, family problems."

D. "You mean your mother-in-law again?"

P. "Oh, my mother-in-law is only part of it really. She isn't really the whole cause. It is not fair to blame it all on her."

D. "No."

P. "I can't say that it is anybody's fault."

D. "Have you felt like this before?"

P. "Oh, yes, badly for about two years."

D. "Yes. You have had help about it before?"

P. "No, not really. This is the first time. (Unable to hear patient, sobbing loudly.) I feel so foolish."

D. "Why do you feel foolish, it is not foolish."

P. "It is so stupid, it is bad to cry and behave like this."

D. "But it isn't. If you can't cry in the surgery, where can you cry?"

P. "Anyway, 1 thought, 1 don't really know what to do. You know it might be all right, I have had this before."

D. "How long has it been so severe as it is now?"

P. "I have had it once before, last year. It has been like this for about two months."

D. "Yes."

P. "But I thought that when I went on holiday it would be all right. You know, that I would get better, because you see I seem to be all right to everybody. Nobody realises this but my husband. I can talk to him and he stopped me. . . . I just don't know. It is partly my husband, but I hate people blaming their husbands for things."

D. "When you say it is partly him, what do you mean?"

P. "Well, it is partly his fault, I think, but I don't know, this is it, it may be my own fault. Years ago my husband was unfaithful to me. But not in the way one talks about being unfaithful today. He took his typist out when we were first married, we were married a very few months at the time, and he didn't have an affair with her, but to me it was a terrible shock."

D. "You felt betrayed by it?"

P. "Oh, yes, because I was very young and I was a very ignorant girl, that's all I can say it was. I thought that people fell in love, got married and lived very pure lives. I was just very ignorant; although I lived in London I led a very sheltered life. I was very ignorant generally of the facts of life. But that

97

was all right, he did that, but I was terrible to him so I can see that it wasn't his fault."

D. "Yes."

P. "Because I was pregnant, I wasn't pregnant when I got married, but I was soon afterwards and I personally was very pleased, but my husband told my parents-in-law, when he came back he said I was to have an abortion."

D. "Yes."

P. "Now to me this was an absolutely terrible thing. I don't think my husband himself wanted it, but he has grown up, you see; it is not fair to talk about somebody when they are young, now they are older and they have changed."

D. "I am sorry to interrupt you, but there is a doctor on the phone."

P. "Yes, certainly."

Telephone call, two minutes.

D. "Now, I am sorry, dear."

P. "That is all right. So that happened anyway his parents, you must remember that I am a Catholic, so to me it was much worse."

D. "Yes, than it might otherwise have been."

P. "I expect, I don't know, people, some people don't mind. But anyhow his parents gave me tablets to take, but anyhow I personally didn't take them, but his parents thought I had taken them. Well, anyway, I didn't have the baby."

D. "You did miscarry or not?"

P. "No. I didn't."

D. "You went on and had the baby?"

P. "Yes. And, of course, everybody was delighted when the baby came."

D. "Yes."

P. "And even afterwards they were very happy, when they knew that it was definite."

D. "You mean, once you got beyond the stage when an abortion was possible?"

P. "Yes. They were quite happy about it and I must say they did everything possible to help us. They were very good to us."

D. "Did you have mixed feelings then? As a result of this conflict?"

P. "Well, you see I always have, this has been the trouble."

D. "Yes."

P. "The point is, I should have by now, have forgotten all this, after all I have been married twenty-three years. So it is about time. . . ."

D. "But your mother-in-law is still living with you."

P. "Yes, has always. Yes. Always there, now my husband, it is sad to say, he loves me very much, but I have never trusted him after that, one hundred per cent. Do you understand?"

D. "Yes. You always had a reservation."

P. "Yes. Always. I was never one hundred per cent. I lost whatever, I suppose happiness, or whatever one has, but through the years I have been happy, we seem to have a very happy, on the surface, a very good marriage. And the children are very happy. But periodically I have over the last few years, I have been getting this terrible black depression. Sometimes it is because my mother-in-law is living with me, and she is going to live with me always. I can see no. . . ."

98

D. "You don't see any end of it, you told me about that before, didn't you, in October?"

P. "Yes, and I don't know, sometimes it seems that it. . . . I mean I have everything, material things, that is all right. I have offered to help with various organisations but they either have too many or they don't need help. And I feel that it is just this kind of black depression, that I just want to die and get rid of . . . just finish with everything. And I know that it is selfish, because of the children."

D. "So you feel guilty about it as well?"

P. "Yes, but not as guilty as I think I should feel, because my husband said I must think of the children."

D. "Please would you tell me a bit more about how you are sleeping?"

P. "Yes. I sleep sometimes for about two to three hours. I waken very early in the morning, about five o'clock. But I did sleep very well last night. I didn't waken until about six-fifteen this morning, so I slept very well. But I hadn't slept the night before. I came yesterday morning, but I hadn't realised that you hadn't got a surgery."

D. "What time did you come?"

P. "I think it was about eleven o'clock. This sleeping is ridiculous, one is very tired."

D. "It isn't ridiculous, it is part of the depression."

P. "Yes, I think it is stupid. . . ."

D. "You are trying to do too much for yourself, at the moment. You can't fight all of this yourself, this is what is called an endogenous depression. It is arising from inside, it may be partly due to being around forty-five."

P. "Yes, yes, of course."

D. "This may have some effect. And it is the sort of thing that responds very well to treatment with tablets. And I think you can look forward to complete recovery and really going back to feeling quite normal again."

P. "Oh, that's grand. Yes."

D. "And being able to cope and all the things that you want to be able to do."

P. "You see I can cope with the housework and I can't stop working. Which is probably very good."

D. "That is your conscience; driving you is it?"

P. "Oh, yes, it is. This is it. But you see there are days when I won't do anything at all. Just go out and sit in the park."

D. "What sort of attitude does your husband take when you are like this? Is he understanding and supporting or . . . ?"

P. "Yes. I would say. But he doesn't quite understand how I feel. But he is, he would do his best."

D. "How can anybody who hasn't been depressed understand exactly how you feel?"

P. "Yes. He is very good I must say."

D. "I have met a lot of people who have been depressed, who have tried to commit suicide, but I still don't quite feel the way they feel, you know. But I do know that this is going to recover. It would recover if we didn't do anything, but we can help it to feel easier now and to get better sooner with some treatment. I would like you to take three tablets during the day and two at night. And I want you to come back and tell me about any problems that you may have. You did say that on Monday when you felt very black you felt like committing suicide; did you have any particular method in mind?"

P. "Yes. I was going to use a razor. But I couldn't find it, because I forgot to put the light on in the bathroom."

D. "What a lucky thing."

P. "And my husband came in, the light was outside the door."

D. "Yes. The other thing is that with depression as severe as this, I do sometimes like to have a second opinion, from a psychiatrist, would you object to this?"

P. "Oh, no. I wouldn't because I want to get better. I want to feel all right, it is stupid to feel like this and very worrying, and I feel I snap at the children."

D. "Yes."

P. "I mean I make a conscious effort not to snap at them, to try and be nice, but I really could shout at them."

D. "Well, you will be able to stop doing that sort of thing within a very short time."

P. "Oh, that is lovely, thank you very much."

D. "I should warn you that treatment of this kind does have some side-effects. And you can expect a rather dry mouth, and perhaps a little blurring of vision in the first few days of treatment. All right? So be prepared for that and don't stop taking the tablets because of that. For the first two days I want you to take three tablets during the day and after that I want you to increase it to what will be labelled."

P. "Yes, for the first two days I take three."

D. "And then two at bedtime, as well, five a day. Please would you make an appointment to see me next Friday?"

P. "I will."

D. "And I am here all the time. If you need somebody in the meantime if you feel as bad as this again then don't hesitate to ring up."

P. "You see, we are newcomers, and our neighbours are very nice, the people have been extremely nice, but I have nobody I can talk to. And what is more, I never feel I can talk to people. I don't like to back-bite my mother-in-law; I will tell you, but I wouldn't dream of telling anybody else."

D. "No, of course not. Well, next week I would like you to tell me a little more about your feelings about your mother-in-law, because she plays an important part in your life, doesn't she?"

P. "Oh, yes, there is no doubt about that."

D. "How old is she?"

P. "She is seventy. But she is a very young seventy. And she is very nice, you see, if she didn't live with me. But I get on very well with her."

D. "But it is at your own personal cost."

P. "Yes, definitely."

(Confused noise.) (End of consultation.)

This is a good example of the style because it contains so little of any other style. It is normal to find that even within a consultation a doctor may use certain behaviours associated with another style. In a discussion about this last example it was suggested to this doctor that he had lots of opportunity to reflect. He recognised this and said that he disliked the reflecting approach because it seemed to him to be too free.

The final example in this chapter is of the very rare "reflecting" style. Its rarity is such that out of more than two thousand consultations not more than fifteen were found to be completely of this style.

D. "Good morning. Sit down. Now then. . . ."
P. "I don't know where to begin."
D. "Mmm. Mmm."
P. "Well, I'm not really ill and I feel a bit of a fraud."
D. "A fraud?"
P. "Well, you are supposed to make me better when I'm ill and I'm not ill."
D. "Mmm. Mmm."
*P. "Well, last week I changed my job."
D. "You changed your job."
P. "Well, I'm not sure what's wrong with me but I think I may have made a mistake."
D. "A mistake?"
P. "Yes, a mistake. I left the other place because we had not enough money. You know my husband has been out of work for a long time. So I changed my job and now I bring in about £5 a week more."
D. "Have you had last week's pay yet?"
P. "Yes, in this place they pay you Monday to Friday and you get it on Friday night."
D. "Today is Tuesday."
*P. "Yes. Well, I took the money home and we're still as broke as ever."
D. "You're broke on Tuesday?"
*P. "Yes. Well, it's difficult. But, well, I give him all the money and then he gives me some for housekeeping."
D. "He gives you some?"
P. "Yes, he gives me £4·50."
D. "Mmm. Mmm."
*P. "Well, there's him and the three kids."
D. "Three kids?"
*P. (Crying.) "It's no good, I can't go on like this. Whatever I earn he will spend. He's not had a proper job in five years. I've had to go out, and have the babies and look after him. And then there's the house."
D. "Mmm. Mmm."
P. "Well, why don't he get a job? What would happen if I get pregnant again? Doctor, I couldn't take it. What will I do?"
D. "Do?"
P. "Yes, when I get pregnant."
D. "Are you pregnant?"
*P. "Oh, God, doctor, I don't know. I don't want to know. Oh, God, I just couldn't do it all over again."
D. "Are you afraid that you are pregnant?"
P. "Well, yes, doctor. You know we don't have any preventions. He won't have it. He says he's a Catholic, but he hasn't been near a church in ten years. He gets drunk on Sunday like any other day. If he gets up in the morning it is only to get his money from the unemployment."
D. "Is there a chance that you are pregnant now? If you like we can check. It won't take long."

P. "Well, that's it. If I am what am I to do?"
D. "What do you want to do?"
P. "Well, I'm afraid to think about it. But I couldn't take time off for that."
D. "For what?"
P. "Well, you know. The operation."

The doctor is now through to a clear understanding of the problem facing the patient. The consultation goes on to examine her fears of an abortion, her religious views and her deteriorating relationship with her husband. During the next interview the patient decided to have an abortion.

The skill in this interview is the way in which the doctor simply reflected the patient's words and enabled her to talk. The other point, which is not obvious from a transcript, is the way in which the doctor refused to break silences. Where a star (*) appears there was a gap of anything up to five or six seconds punctuating the patient's replies. Any attempt by the doctor to hasten the interview by probing or even making assumptions would probably have been counter-productive.

As has been stated, the majority of consultations are normally a mixture of "gathering information" and "analysing and probing". There are a few occasions when a style is used which is not covered by these two descriptions. The following example was provided by a doctor who would normally be described as an "analysing prober". In this particular case his performance was rather different.

D. "Good morning. Sit down. What can I do for you today?"
P. "Well, I think I've got the 'flu, doctor."
D. "Well, there's not much of it about now."
P. "Well, I've got this cold. . . ."
D. "Yes. I can see that. Shivering a bit, are you?"
P. "Yes."
D. "Mmm. Well, there's not a lot to worry about is there? Now you take this to the chemist and you'll be all right in three or four days."

In this particular case the doctor very nearly was a party to a minor catastrophe. The patient subsequently was diagnosed as suffering from pleurisy. This evidence was offered freely by the doctor, who was suffering far more from his poor performance than the patient. He admitted that he had not conducted any sort of examination and was predisposed towards the diagnosis of common cold when he saw the patient blowing his nose as he entered the consulting-room.

His reasoning was quite interesting. This patient was the last of 26 in a crowded morning surgery. He had appeared without an appointment just before the doctor was due to leave on his morning calls. The doctor was already 30 minutes late for his first home visit. Nine of his previous patients had also suffered from "common colds". He therefore "assumed" that the patient was exaggerating his condition and acted upon that assumption.

It is worth noting that styles do change during a full surgery. With the best will in the world a doctor cannot keep up clarifying or reflecting through 25 patients in a morning surgery. Surgeries which are crowded have one interesting characteristic. The consultations get shorter as the time wears on. It is very difficult to have a reflective consultation in 30 seconds.

The four basic diagnostic styles have been related to the behaviours identified in Chapters 4 to 7. In order to do this a set of consultations was selected which appeared to have dominant styles. The most common behaviours were then listed.

Figure 2

USE OF PATIENTS KNOWLEDGE AND EXPERIENCE			USE OF DOCTORS SPECIAL SKILL AND KNOWLEDGE
SILENCE LISTENING REFLECTING	CLARIFYING & INTERPRETING	ANALYSING & PROBING	GATHERING INFORMATION
Offering observation	Broad question	Direct question	Direct question
Encouraging	Clarifying	Correlational question	Closed question
Clarifying	Challenging	Placing events	Correlational question
Reflecting	Repeating for affirmation	Repeating for affirmation	Placing events
Using patient ideas.	Seeking patient idea	Suggesting	Summarising to close off
Seeking patient ideas	Offering observation	Offering feeling	Suggesting
Indicating understanding.	Concealed question	Exploring	Self answering questions
Using silence	Placing events	Broad question.	Reassuring
	Summarising to open up.		Repeating for affirmation
			Justifying self chastising

It must be emphasised that no doctor follows a particular style with any rigidity, but most tend to operate within two styles. Thus, a doctor who prefers to "gather information" will also be able to "analyse and probe". He will, however, show little evidence of any ability to move right across the range of styles to "reflecting". Equally, doctors who prefer to reflect show little interest in gathering information except when working under pressure of time. Another cause of a doctor moving his style in order to gather information is frequently an immigrant patient (or family) and the equally frequent language difficulty.

Some doctors have claimed that they alter their style in the same fashion to cope with British patients who display a limited verbal ability. From the evidence we have on tape this is not true. What they appear to do is to ask the same questions in the same way only more slowly and occasionally more loudly.

CHAPTER 10
DOCTORS AND CONSULTING STYLES: GROUPING BEHAVIOURS (PART II)

In the last chapter we concerned ourselves with the ways in which a doctor might proceed in a consultation to that point where he makes some sort of

103

decision about the condition of the patient. We itemised four basic styles which appear to constitute a spectrum. To make the analysis we used a model familiar to students of social psychology in which the balance of power between two parties in any given activity is diagrammatically represented by a simple model.

In this chapter we will use the same model and the same components, viz the doctor's skill and knowledge and the patient's experience and knowledge. There is a complication in this model because we discovered that whilst a spectrum of four basic styles adequately explained the diagnostic phases of a consultation, the same four styles are inadequate to explain the prescriptive phases. Originally we tried to compress all our findings into four styles, but this only served to demonstrate that such a spectrum was inadequate to cover the range we were now concerned with. After various experiments we found that a range encompassing seven styles was the basic minimum we could use.

This in itself is not a startling and significant finding. Doctors are aware that even the clearest of diagnoses do not necessarily have single and unique forms of treatment. Furthermore, even a relatively simple piece of direction contains two basic elements—what the doctor has to do for the patient and what the patient has to do for himself. Take the simplest example of all:

"Take this to the chemist. Take the tablets three times daily after meals."

By prescribing a programme of medication the doctor is playing his part. The patient has still to be committed to playing his part by going to the chemist and by subsequently following the routine laid down for him by the doctor. How the doctor secures the commitment of the patient to that routine is a matter of wide choice.

The tapes we have analysed contain, inevitably, a large number of consultations in which the diagnosis was "infection of the upper respiratory tract". If we assume that doctors do see this condition very frequently and we assume that the diagnosis is probably correct we can begin our analysis of prescribing behaviour by examining just what doctors do when dealing with such cases. In addition to the direction issued in the example above we have also heard the following:

(a) "You have an infection of the upper respiratory tract. More likely than not it will clear itself in three or four days. This prescription may well clear it faster."

(b) "Take this to the chemist. Come back next week if it is not better."

(c) "You have a little infection at the back there. Do you want a prescription?"

(d) "Now then, I am going to give you some tablets for this. It's just a little infection. I want you to take these every six hours. Now then, not like last time. I want you to take them all until the bottle is finished. Okay?"

The diagnosis in each case is the same. What happens subsequently is a matter of judgement in which the doctor is deciding how to cope with both the infection and the patient.

Let us now examine a rather different situation. In the next two extracts we are concerned with patients who are recovering from coronary thromboses. The crises periods are now receding into the past and the doctor in each case is concerned to progress the gradual rehabilitation of the patients. Both patients are male in their mid-forties. In both cases the doctor has completed his physical examination which was accompanied by a verbal examination.

Case 1

D. "Okay, put your shirt back on, please. Now then, I think it is time that you went back to work. However, I think that you must only go back for a few hours a day and at the least sign of tiredness you must stop. I don't want you smoking any more and you are not under any circumstances to take any form of strong liquor. You will stay on all of the tablets for the time being and we will start to reduce the dosage next month. You are not to drive. You're not driving are you?"

P. "No. The wife brought me here today."

D. "Good. Let's keep it like that for the time being, shall we?"

Case 2

D. "Well, now, Mr—— you seem to be making a reasonable recovery. How did you get here today?"

P. "Oh. I came on foot."

D. "Mmm. Mmm. How did it feel?"

P. "Out of breath two or three times but I rested."

D. "Splendid. Well, that's something you can slowly expect to build up. But whilst you need some exercise you must take it very carefully."

P. "What about work, doctor?"

D. "Well, how do you feel about it?"

P. "Well, I think I could manage a few hours a day, you know."

D. "Mmm. Mmm. How will you get there?"

P. "My neighbour works in the same office. He could take me."

D. "Mmm. Mmm. Well, I don't want you in there for too long at first."

P. "You mean I should stay away?"

D. "No. I think you must decide when you go back. If you think you can manage now, then it's fine. But two or three hours is enough."

P. "Well, I'll make a try next Monday."

D. "Okay. Let's look at how you are eating. How's the diet going?"

P. "No trouble, but it's rather boring."

As can be seen, the same route is being followed but in a rather different fashion. The first doctor is laying down clear instructions and is allowing the patient to play little part in the activity. The second doctor is more concerned to find out how the patient thinks he is progressing and is encouraging him to accept some responsibility for his action.

This, of course, is what doctors claim they do. They believe that they match their patterns of prescribing to the patient and his condition. In fact, such evidence as we have suggests that doctors have a fairly standard method of closing any consultation which in our terms has a consistent placing on the doctor/patient centred scale.

In the previous chapter we observed that doctors may well move across two of the styles with reasonable ease but only rarely did they move across three styles. In this chapter we have already indicated we are dealing with seven styles and our observations suggest that a range of three of these styles describes the ability of the vast majority of doctors. Furthermore, as we noted in the previous chapter, the styles used by any particular doctor will normally lie together on the spectrum. There are, however, a few notable exceptions. As we will observe in our examination of Style 6, this style was observed to be used on a number of occasions by doctors who normally use Styles 1 or 2. In these cases it was used as a reserve style when the preferred style appeared to have failed.

Figure 3

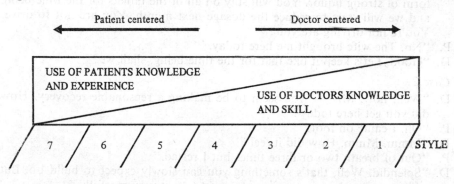

Style 1. The most extreme form of doctor behaviour after the completion of the diagnosis might be described as follows: *Doctor makes a decision about the patient and his treatment and then instructs the patient to seek some service.* This is a most common finish to a consultation. The doctor completes his examination of the patient and then uses a word form such as below:

> "Well, now, take this along to the chemist. Take them three times daily after meals. 'Bye-bye"

or

> "I'll make an appointment for you to have an X-ray. Now don't worry. We'll be in touch. Cheerio."

This style tells the patient absolutely nothing about his condition but does indicate that something is wrong if only because consequent actions have to be taken. In terms of Chapter 6 these doctors end their consultations with "direction" and "direct termination". In terms of Chapter 5 there is no Phase IV and only the barest Phase V. It is a rapid means of terminating a consultation and occurs in some form or other in 624 of the 2,000+ cases we analysed.

Style 2. *The doctor makes his decision and announces it*

For example:

> "Well now, you seem to have nothing more than a bout of influenza. Take this to the chemist on your way home. Go to bed for a few days and I'll look in from time to time. Okay? Good. Off you go now"

or

> "This is an infection of the lung. I want you to go upstairs and have an X-ray now. When you have had that come back here and I will detail more treatment."

These are strong endings to consultations, but they differ from Style 1 in so far as the doctor does at least tell the patient what is causing the suffering. They are also terminating in that there is little room for the patient to do anything but agree.

106

In this style typical behaviour units are:

Giving information
Directing
Terminating.

Again this is a very common way of completing a consultation. Somewhat more common than the previous style, it occurs 680 times.

Style 3. *The doctor sells his decision to the patient*

There are very few examples of the doctors actually selling to the patient, and most of the examples come from one doctor who appears to use it as his primary prescribing style.

"Now then, Mrs T——, you've got the same again. Now then, I would like you to take this prescription along to the chemist. Now then, how do you feel about that? No, don't worry, it's no more serious than it was last time. Yes, it's just the same as before. Okay, my dear? Right then, off you go. Cheeribye."

This does indeed sound like a soap salesman using a common selling model. The patient does not make a sound during the whole performance. There may well have been non-verbal cues which triggered off parts of the whole, but it still has the character of selling about it. This type of termination is also a strong way to finish a consultation because the patient plays such a little part. The behaviour units used are a mixture of:

Giving information
Directing
Reassuring
Seeking patient ideas (but not using them)
Direct termination.

This style of concluding only occurs on its own in 57 consultations. It is used as a back-up strategy in another 70 cases and is found mainly in consultations by "reassuring" doctors. It has some of the style of a much more permissive termination of a consultation. Its real effect, however, is to close just as firmly as any of the two previous styles.

These first three styles of closure contain very little of what has been described as Phase IV behaviour. As closing styles, they are commonly used by doctors who begin a consultation with "information gathering". Also these styles of closure are found, but with a much lower frequency, in doctors who normally use much more open endings (see Styles 5, 6 and 7), but who for various reasons find themselves subject to time pressures. (See Conclusions.)

Style 4. *The doctor presents a tentative decision subject to change*

For example:

"Now then, you appear to be having some more trouble with that leg of yours. This is, I think, a consequence of the fact that you are still trying to work as you did ten years ago. Now you are fifty-five and you really ought to start taking things a little easier. I think you ought to have a long rest. Now then, how do you think you can cope with that?"

This style differs from the previous styles in that it involves the patient marginally in his own treatment. It also indicates that the doctor is, to some degree, willing to amend his plan for the management of the patient.

107

For example:

P. "Well, I'm not sure that I can stop work for the next two weeks. You see, the wife isn't working at the moment, and we won't be able to live without my pay."

D. "Okay. In that case we will have to consider deferring your rest until then. In the meanwhile I want you to try and take things more easily at work."

In this particular style the doctor has a limited number of strategies in mind for the patient, but is trying his preferred strategy first. The final decision partly rests with the patient. This style is very often used when dealing with patients who must change their work or life-style. Most doctors recognise that changes of this sort cannot be made simply by telling the patient to do something. Therefore, a degree of choice and a desire for consensus is required. This style was observed in 92 consultations.

A variation on this style might be described as follows:

"The doctor presents his decision and invites questions."

This definition sounds rather more authoritarian than our previous definition. The end product of the questioning is often a modification of the decisions in the light of patient's opinion. This variant does have an apparent weakness in that it occasionally degenerates into an "I will if you will" situation.

For example:

D. "This condition is caused by your smoking. I want you to give up smoking at once. No more cigarettes, do you see? I want you to stop now. Do you understand what I mean?"

P. "Well, doctor, it's not that easy is it?"

D. "Well, I can't continue to treat you if you keep on smoking in this way."

P. "Well, I can try to cut it down, but can't you give me some tablets to help?"

D. "I don't place much faith in tablets. All you have to do is to stop."

P. "But you can't stop just like that, can you?"

D. "Well, you can buy those tablets at any chemist."

P. "Can't you give me a prescription for them?"

And so on.

Typical behaviours of Style 4 are:

Giving information or opinion
Directing
Advising
Answering patient questions
Seeking patient ideas
Indicating understanding
Using patient ideas.

This version of Style 4 conclusion was observed in 279 consultations.

Style 5. *The doctor presents the problem, seeks suggestions and makes decisions*

In some ways this is a variable style, because although it sounds more consultative than the previous style, it can still conclude with a very strong termination.

For example:

D. "Your condition is probably worse than when I last examined you. Now then, in the first place you are going to have to stop lifting those bags of cement."

P. "But doctor, I don't have any other sort of work."

108

D. "What other work have you thought of?"
P. "Well, I might get a job driving a van."
D. "Have you tried to get a job driving a van?"
P. "Well, yes, but at my age no one will look at me."
D. "Have you been down to the Labour Exchange?"
P. "Well, no. I mean, you don't go down there when you have a job do you?"
D. "Who told you that?"
P. "Well, nobody. But I've always thought that."
D. "Right. Well now. Tomorrow morning you go to the Labour Exchange. See if you can get a job doing something light. If you like I'll write a note for you as well. Oh, and take this to the chemist on your way home. Okay? 'Bye-bye."

This doctor used the patient's suggestion about van driving to enable him to clarify his own ideas about patient management. Yet the doctor is still making the decision for the patient, and in this particular case without any real examination of the implications. What transpired was that the patient returned a day later to confront the doctor with the relative difference in wages for van driving and heavy labouring.

This particular interview, which was discussed at length with the GP concerned and a group of 16 other GPs, produced an insight into the insensitivity of some GPs to the effects and consequences of their decisions. All GPs are familiar with the consequences of what might be termed "medical decision making". They are well aware of most of the effects of chemotherapy, and of the effects of such treatment as surgery. They display, in some cases, however, a lack of insight into the real consequences of advising a patient to change his life style. Prescribing a change of life style is infinitely more threatening to the patient than is the prescribing of medicines, yet, judging from the tapes, few doctors bother to go into detail with the patient about how the latter might accommodate to the proposed change. In terms of cold statistics it must be added that the average doctor prevents himself from undertaking such an activity anyway. As an average consultation lasts for about $5\frac{1}{2}$ minutes, and the average diagnosis seems to occur at around 3 minutes, the $2\frac{1}{2}$ minutes left is little indeed in which to discuss the problems of the patient changing his life style.

The group of GPs which discussed the last consultation was badly split over this issue. Such comments were made as:

"If we were to do all that we would never finish our surgeries"

or

"We cannot accept this degree of responsibility for all our patients"

or

"Our job is simply to confront the patient with his choice. He, however, must make the choice."

Others in the same group took the view that such decisions, if badly made, have the effect of causing the patient to reappear in the surgery week after week, and thus use up just as much time, but spread out over a long period.

Typical behaviours of Style 5 are:

Giving information or opinion

Advising

Clarifying
Reflecting
Exploring
Seeking patient ideas
Using patient ideas
Offering collaboration
Terminating (indirect).

This style was observed in 159 cases.

Style 6. *The doctor defines the limits and requests the patient to make a decision*

For example:

"Now then, this condition is no more than a simple appendicitis. It can be quickly treated by surgery, although at this stage that is not the best possible answer. I can also treat you at home with some drugs. This treatment will take a short time if you rest. If you have to keep working then the treatment will take rather longer, and may not be so effective. The choice is yours."

Style 6 occurs either as the doctor's primary strategy (35 instances), in which case he will help the patient to evaluate the choices; or it occurs with doctors who have failed with Styles 1 or 2 (39 instances). In the latter case, as soon as the patient makes a choice, the doctor accepts and terminates.

As a reserve style for 1 or 2 it is not of much interest, but as a pure style it does produce interesting interchanges between doctor and patient. In the above example the following interchange took place after the piece of consultation already quoted:

P. "Why do you say that an operation is not really the best course of action?"
D. "Well, you know, medical opinion can be a terribly fickle thing. Years ago we would have had it out by now. But the introduction of things like antibiotics has meant that some of these infections can be contained and controlled. Given what you have, I don't think I would advise an operation if I were your surgeon."
P. "Fine, what about treating me at home?"
D. "Well, that is my ideal treatment at this stage. If you can rest for a few days, and take the various prescriptions, I think we will clear this thing up."
P. "But will it come back?"
D. "Well, it might, because nothing is certain. It is not uncommon now to treat this in this way. It is also much less traumatic than surgery."
P. "Well, I don't like the idea of going to work, so I think I'll go home, go to bed with a few good books and let you fill me full of drugs."
D. "Fine. Okay. Hang on. I've got a few tablets in this drawer. That'll save a prescription. If they work I'll let you have some more. I'll call in at your house tonight and then again tomorrow. Okay? Now then, don't run. In fact take a taxi. 'Bye."

This style is also quite common, occurring 74 times. The doctor is still well in control of the situation, but, having spelled out all the alternatives, is then quite prepared to accept whichever of them the patient cares to select. It is clearly not a style relevant to a critical condition, but it can be used when the doctor has a number of options open to him.

110

Typical behaviours of Style 6 are:
  Giving information
  Answering patient questions
  Seeking patient ideas
  Using patient ideas
  Summarising to open up
  Pre-directional probing.

Style 7. *The doctor permits the patient to make his own decision*

This is a very rare style and only occurs in a very limited number of situations (22 cases). A group of GPs applied two quite different definitions to it. One group decided it was the "ideal style for the management of the hypochondriac", whilst another group decided it was the style for the doctor who "was faced with some sort of emotional problem and did not know what to do with it".

For example:

"Now then, Mrs T——, we have got to the point where we know that you have been to see the specialist three times. On each occasion he has sent me a negative report. We have been in hospital for observation twice and on each occasion we have drawn a blank. Now here you are again with the same symptoms, and I accept that for you the pain is real so we must accept it as real. I've run a full examination and, apart from your blood pressure being a little high, I can find nothing wrong. Your X-ray plates are back and they are clean. But as you say, you still feel ill, and this makes you depressed. Most of what I do for you only produces temporary results. My opinion is that this is what we call a psychosomatic illness and we now have to find out what causes it. Now then, what I want you to think about is what we should do next."

A better example is as follows:
D. "Well now, this is your heart you know, how do you feel about that?"
P. "Do you think I ought to stop work?"
D. "How would you feel about that?"
P. "Well, I think it would make me a lot better."
D. "Mmm. Mmm."
P. "I could take a few weeks off and rest you know."
D. "Does the idea appeal to you?"
P. "Yes. I know that I am under a lot of strain. And I knew all along what you were going to tell me here. I know I've got to have a rest. I've closed my eyes to the fact that those tablets are for the angina."
D. "So you knew all along?"
P. "Yes, doctor. Let's face it. I'm sixty-nine. I should have retired years ago. But I've no interests except work. It's time now to have a rest."

This style seems to be a natural consequence of a reflective Phase II and III but occurs with much less frequency than the reflective diagnostic interview. Many GPs will occasionally use reflection as an end to achieving a diagnosis, but then follow up with something like Style 4 or 5. When questioned about this many GPs have indicated a reticence about Style 7 because they fear the risks which its use might involve.

"It's okay allowing the patient to help you make a diagnosis, but in the last resort you are there to prescribe. If you fail in that, then you are in trouble."

111

Typical behaviours of Style 7 are:
  Reflecting
  Encouraging
  Seeking patient ideas
  Using patient ideas.

CHAPTER 11

DISCUSSION OF "DOCTORS' STYLES" IN THE CONSULTATION

The question needs to be asked, "How do these styles come to be formed?" What is remarkable, as we shall show, is the consistency of style shown by doctors. Within the normal range of patients seen in a series of morning and evening surgeries, one would expect to find a range of illness running from the purely organic through to the more difficult to determine psychosomatic. Equally, one would expect (and in fact does find) a range of patients with considerable differences in verbal ability. We have not been able to examine social class differences because so many urban practices have a limited class range of patients.

While the patient's input into the consultation contains a wide range of variables it is surprising to discover that the individual doctor's responses are standardised to a remarkable degree.

Some of the explanation must lie in the ways in which doctors have learned to consult with patients. Despite a considerable volume of literature which appears to emphasise the importance of the consultation there is not extant a formal system of training in the skills of consulting. It is something that a doctor is expected to pick up as he progresses through his training. It is also true to observe that most educational systems fight shy of attempting any training in the consultation because of the assumed difficulty in deciding what has to be learned.

A doctor then formulates his own consultation behaviour from his potential models during a range of experiences starting with his own family GP, his teachers in hospital and medical school, possibly a parent or relative in medicine, or (at worst) a few televisual fantasies. As a result, the learning of consulting skills is casual, experiential and assisted by trial and error.

By the time a GP gets into his own surgery, unless he has been processed through one of the better of the new training schemes, he is largely dependent upon a limited range of experience, most of which is probably derived from a hospital setting.

This research was not intended to cover consultants, or the various specialised disciplines of medicine, but a few consultants have provided short periods of taped consultation. The following transcript is of a consultant cardiologist dealing with a referral. A great deal of this consultation, which lasted for seven minutes, is just noise as the consultant attaches the patient to a machine and conducts a series of routine tests. It would be tempting to state that few GPs would be able to work successfully with the degree of insensitivity displayed in

112

the second half of this consultation. The truth is that many GPs are capable of emulating this performance.

D. "Come in. Now then, Mr Z——. You have been sent to me by Dr G——. Good. Now then, just settle in over there and I'll refresh my memory."

P. "Thank you, sir."

D. "Ah, yes. Fine. Would you take your clothes off to the waist please?"

P. "Yes, of course."

D. "Now then, let's have a little check. Breathe. Good. Breathe. Good. Now then, sit down here a minute will you?"

P. "Yes."

D. "Right you are. Now then, this machine does a few tests for me. Just don't look at it if it frightens you. I'll just attach it. Here you see. Good. Here. Good. Right now. Just carry on breathing normally. Don't get nervous. Have you had a blood test yet?"

P. "Yes, sir."

D. "Oh, yes. Here's the report. Mmm. Mmm. Now then. Excellent. Now then. I'll write to Dr G——. He'll have all the information."

P. "But is anything wrong, sir?"

D. "Well, it's not for me to say, but I think that you'll find the news is not all bad."

P. "Will I have to go into hospital?"

D. "Well, that's up to your Dr G—— really. I can only advise him. Let's see what he has to say. Right you are. Good-bye."

In fairness it should be added that this consultant can be defended in his refusal to divulge information, even though it is an over-zealous adherence to medical niceties. Any GP behaving in such a fashion has no such excuse. Yet, despite this, many GPs do approach consultations in this way. No GP can be quite so negative about the condition of the patient, but nearly a quarter of our sample conducted consultations similar to the one below:

    (Dr L ——.)

D. "Now then, you are Mr W—— of. . . . What is the trouble?"

P. "Well, I feel tired although I'm getting plenty of sleep."

D. "Tired, all the time?"

P. "Last night I went to bed about twelve and I didn't get up until about twelve today because I'm on night work, and it was a struggle getting out of bed, and all day I've had to try and make myself do something, I just wondered. . . ."

D. "Are you sleeping all right?"

P. "Well, I seem to be."

D. "Seem to be. Are you tired first thing in the morning when you wake up?"

P. "Yes."

D. "It might be that you are not sleeping properly, it might not be deep enough. What's your job?"

P. "A stereotyper."

D. "And what time do you work?"

P. "Eight o'clock until half-past three, eight at night until half-past three in the morning."

D. "And you get home about—fourish?"

P. "I go to bed straight away."

D. "And sleep for how long?"

P. "About eleven o'clock."

D. "And you're at home during the day-time?"

P. "I wake up sometimes about half-past seven when the kiddies are getting up for school but I go right back off again."

The doctor has now made his decision on the basis of the information he has gained through his fairly direct questioning of the patient. The only insight he has offered the patient could well have been derived from a Horlicks advertisement:

"It might be that you are not sleeping properly, it might not be deep enough."

What happens next is quite astonishing in its swiftness.

D. "Take one tablet when you go to bed . . . whether you need them or you don't need them, take them and see me in a fortnight, all right? And I'm giving you some capsules. Take one of them every day and let me know what happens in a fortnight."

P. "Very good."

To demonstrate the consistency of this particular doctor a further short example is included. This one is nearly unique because we have met the patient before in Chapter 9. On that occasion the child was alone and asking for an X-ray. In this particular case the child and mother appear together in the partner's surgery because the "normal" doctor was on holiday.

P. "Well, he's been coming in with his cough, doctor."

D. "It was clear last time."

P. "Yes, but he's still coughing a bit."

D. "What about breathing?"

P. "Well, he's wheezing a bit, not now, but he's still coughing."

D. "And he's taking a tablet at night?"

P. "Well, he's taking them twice a day. . . ."

D. "Oh, twice a day, I'm sorry."

P. "I've got two tablets left."

D. "How bad is the cough still?"

P. "Well, it's annoying, still annoying him."

D. "Night or day?"

P. "You cough at school, don't you?"

D. "Coughs at school. . . ."

P. "They don't seem to notice. . . ."

D. "Well, I'll put him on to this medicine, all right? Two spoons night and day, all right?"

P. "Yes."

D. "Bring him back in a fortnight and we'll see how he is."

P. "He's got an ulcer in his mouth, would you have a look at it?"

D. "How much does it trouble you?"

P. (Child.) "A lot."

D. "Get some plain peanuts, or cashew nuts, not salted, plain, and after he has chewed them let him put his tongue over that and chew this. Right?"

P. "Right, thank you."

114

D. "See you in a fortnight's time. 'Bye-bye."

Note that once again this doctor does not give the parent the slightest insight into what might be wrong with the child. The only diagnostic information offered on this occasion is by the mother, who says that the child has an ulcer in his mouth.

The fact that so many doctors conduct this sort of consultation suggests that there must be something upon which the standardised model has been based. We are not suggesting that the consultation involving the consultant cardiologist is necessarily typical of all consultants, but there is a distinct similarity between that consultation and at least 20 per cent of GP consultations.

One of the very real problems with these doctor-centred consulting styles is the way in which the doctor becomes himself a victim of the style and displays a remarkable inability to cope with anything but the most mechanical relationship with the patient.

The next example is Dr R——, who has already been the subject of two consultations in Chapter 9. This particular consultation was the subject of an analysis conducted by six other doctors on a training programme in 1973. Dr R—— had the misfortune to find himself in a sub-group of doctors containing two Balint-trained members. Some of the comments they made at the time are included as a commentary on this consultation. It is also probably true that at least 30 per cent of the medical profession would consider his performance as adequate.

The patient is new to the doctor and to the locality. As will be seen she is not short of problems in her recent past but did sound quite remarkably composed when she started to speak.

(Dr R—— II.)

D. "Hello, come and sit down. Mrs J——? New patient?"
P. "Yes, of Dr S——, from B. . . ."
D. "What is your address?"
P. "M—— Street."
D. "That's Salford, and your date of birth?"
P. "Tenth of October, nineteen forty-five."
D. "Have you given your card to the . . .?"
P. "Yes, I have."
D. "What's the trouble?"
P. "Well, I've been attending Dr S—— for my nerves, I've just been recently separated and my home has been sold at B——, and also I've just had a breast growth removed, which has caused me some anxiety."
D. "Did they just take the lump? Or the whole breast?"
P. "No, just the lump."
D. "Who did that?"
P. "It was at the Northern, Dr B——."
D. "Have you had the report?"
P. "Yes, it was fibroid."
D. "That's okay then. Is he seeing you again?"
P. "I have been back and am being discharged."
D. "When was that done, the operation?"
P. "Six weeks ago. I've just gone back to work."

At this point one of the doctors listening to this tape commented that he was in danger of losing sight of the fact that the most significant things she had said so far were "growth" and "anxiety".

D. "And what are you on for your nerves?"

P. "I keep having very bad dreams every night since we've split up and I've brought these to show you what he's been giving me, but I've still been having these bad dreams and I've been having these three times a day."

D. "Do these seem to help?"

P. "Well, I don't really know. Well, obviously, they must do."

This produced a reaction in the listening group who felt that this response was so evasive and transparent that the doctor would be very insensitive not to follow it up.

D. "Have you any children?"

P. "No."

D. "Is it hard since you've split up?"

P. "Well, it's hard on his part, yes."

The doctor admitted that he had no idea what the patient meant by this, and again was taxed by his group for not dealing with her evasion.

D. "How long have you been married?"

P. "Six years."

D. "It's very upsetting."

P. "Yes, very."

D. ". . . It's surprising how things can change, even in a few weeks. How long have you been separated?"

P. "Well, we've been separated since August, but our home's only been split for about five weeks. . . ."

The patient is now about to start talking about something and must have given the doctor some non-verbal cues as well because he interrupts her.

D. "Well, I will give you something to sleep and something to calm you down, and if these suit you we'll keep you on those but I think we'll change the. . . . Do you feel it helps?"

P. "Yes, I do really. Obviously, I was very worried about this lump as well. . . ."

The patient has made one final attempt to say something to the doctor, but from now on there is no possible way in which the doctor is going to allow her to expose him to her fears. At every opportunity he talks. Notice how much more of the consultation he now occupies. The patient is reduced to a series of "yesses" culminating in a very depressing, "Thank you very much indeed".

D. "Mogadon?"

P. "Yes."

D. "And instead of these Mogadon we'll just give you a capsule to take. This will help you to sleep. It isn't a sleeping capsule but it will help you to sleep, but it will also work during the day to try and lift this depression."

P. "Yes."

D. "Now I'm just going to give you enough for two weeks and I will want to see you again then."

P. "Yes."

D. "Have they given you a surgery card with the hours and the appointments system? This is the card. It's got the doctors' names and surgery hours and the various . . . and the telephone numbers and so on."

116

P. "Thank you very much indeed."

D. "Now I will see you again in two weeks. With all these nerve tablets, they take about ten days before you get any effect—so don't expect a lot. About a week or ten days. By the time you come back you should notice a difference. Right, see you in a fortnight and see what happens."

All of the doctors we have studied in this chapter have busy city practices and appear to average one patient every five minutes. They claim, perhaps with some justification, that they could not manage their practices unless they maintain this sort of rate. Perforce in this study we have examined this doctor-centred style at length. From this study a number of factors were identified as being associated with the style. As noted above, the busy practice is always there. Secondly, there is a distinct preference by the doctor for the treatment of the first symptoms offered. Thirdly, and perhaps most important, there is an apparent inability or unwillingness to enter into any real relationship with patients. This is made very apparent by the way in which these doctors prevent and stifle any expression of feeling in the consultation. Throughout the interviews there is an apparent desire to maintain their relationships with patients almost on a technocratic basis. One may even suspect that these very impersonal styles are defence mechanisms which protect doctors against patients.

These three factors have been identified by several of the members of courses as being both an essential part and the basic problem of general practice. Sadly, there is a sort of "catch 22" implicit in all their arguments. You cannot afford to spend too much time looking for deep-seated problems in patients because too many patients keep coming back all the time for more treatment.

It is clear that a doctor with the sort of style we have been examining so far will not be very much use to patients who have psychosomatic problems or even those who have difficulty in talking about their problems. We must, at the same time, admit that nothing in our study suggests that for most physiological disorders afflicting reasonably articulate patients the style can be bettered.

We are now going to look at two more consultations, this time conducted by a doctor who freely admitted, before coming on a training programme, that he was "all at sea with psychosocial problems". If we examine his style we will see that he is not simply a gatherer of information. He goes further and explores and suggests. He is not an exponent of either of the two patient-centred styles of diagnosis.

His first consultation is a good example of how he approaches a physiological problem. Other doctors considered that his performance as a clinician in this consultation was very good. He is certainly thorough, spending nearly nine minutes with the patient. He normally plans his surgeries on the basis of seven patients per hour, thus allocating at least eight minutes to a patient.

(Dr B——.)

D. "Good morning. Come in. Take a seat."

P. "It is the same thing as last year. It is not as bad as last year. . . ."

D. "Just remind me then what was it that was your chief complaint."

P. "Lumbago, I think. You remember, I got examined. . . ."

D. "Yes, I remember. Now where is the pain worst of all?"

P. "It is just round about my hip, and it goes right down my leg. Last night, that leg I had to drag it up the stairs."

D. "Does it go down the front or the back of your leg?"

P. "It goes down the front, here, down below the knee."

D. "How long have you had it this time for?"

P. "Friday it started. This leg bothered me last week, I lost a day off work. And this one started on Friday with my back. I think it's the cold."

D. "It just tends to come in cold weather?"

P. "Yes."

D. "And you had the same pains in your right knee last week?"

P. "No. This one sort of swelled last week."

D. "I see. Do you get any aches and pains anywhere else apart from your back and knees?"

P. "Well . . . on my joints. You see I worked eight years or more down the pit and I just put it down to this. Last year was the worst I have had."

D. "When you get these aches and pains, do they come at any particular time of day?"

P. "My back persists from early morning. And it is just a dull ache, you know. It is here all the time and it seems to travel down my leg to my knee."

D. "How are you in the mornings, putting your boots on?"

P. "Not too bad."

D. "Or putting your briefs on in the morning?"

P. "Okay."

D. "Are you stiff in the back when that happens?"

P. "Sometimes. But last year it started as it is now and I couldn't even move in bed."

D. "Yes, I remember it last year. And you say also, stiffness in fingers and hands."

P. "If I lie on them. I often get up, my hands are dead. They are limp, you have got to use a hand to lift one up."

D. "Is this just through lying on them or can it happen even if you are not lying on them?"

P. "It is hard to say. I can get it quite often."

D. "Do you get any swelling of your fingers or knuckles?"

P. "No."

D. "Wrists or elbows?"

P. "No."

D. "And how long is the longest these aches and pains last in each joint?"

P. "Well, I had this one for about a fortnight. I think I lost a day off work. I think I came down for a line, and they don't give out lines, a doctor's certificate, they don't give out doctor's certificates unless you have been off three days, and I was only off the one day, you see."

D. "I see. So it lasted two weeks in that joint. Do they ever come and go within a couple of days?"

P. "Yes."

D. "Have you been doing more recently, lifting, bending, stooping?"

P. "Well, you see the site is in a terrible state and you have to go up and down, up and down, and it is hard, if you have something wrong with your legs. The cold, the basin we call it, it is pretty hard."

D. "You are doing a lot of walking over rocks and things."

P. "I walk all the time, and I am out in it all the time, standing."

118

D. "I see. And if you have been doing a lot of walking do you find that your ankles give way at all? Or your knees give way on you?"

P. "No. My knees, that is the only part that bothers me. When the pain isn't there I am as fit as anybody else."

D. "Is there anyone in your family with any joint trouble?"

P. "My father, he is dead now, he had acute arthritis."

D. "And how old was he when he began to get trouble with his joints?"

P. "I would reckon about the same as me, thirty-five or thirty-six. He was in a plaster cast and he got small bones broken in his wrists. . . ."

D. "And how have you been feeling generally? Appetite, energy, weight?"

P. "Okay."

D. "You are all right, it is just your joints. Well, we had better have a look at this back again. Can you pop through to the little room."

Tape continues after examination.

D. "Well now, there are no finding of arthritis or joint changes or anything like that. But you have got these tender spots on your elbow and the back of your neck between your shoulders. And I am sure this is right, it is contributed to by the weather, your work and the working in the wet. And having to bend and stoop a lot. This is not the arthritis that your father had."

P. "The sciatica."

D. "You haven't got sciatica, in fact, but I think in the present weather conditions you ought to take a week off your work. And to give your body a chance to supple up again. Now, what do you think about that?"

P. "That would do me fine. I would like to, I have been having trouble with my ears as well. I was in agony for a fortnight with my ears, both ears. You see, we are up high in the wind, I try to get protection clothing over here."

D. "Well, I think you stand a good deal and you should get protective clothing, in your job."

P. ". . . but he wouldn't give me it."

D. "Well, I will give you a doctor's line then. I will give it to you because you sound as if your job needs it. Now, in the meantime you take these tablets, two twice a day and two at night. And take them until you have finished the course for ten days. And here is a line to keep you off for this week. Now, assuming that you have no complaints on Monday, then go back to work again. Now you say you need a medical line for clothing, well, I'll give you a medical line for clothing and this will enable you to get it from the employer."

P. "Well, if I ask him and he refuses, shall I come back to you?"

D. "Well, come back to me. Now we will do these investigations on you and these will take about a week to come back, these blood tests, and I think if you could come in about a week's time for the results of them. And we will explain the result to you then. But there is nothing to be unduly alarmed about, I think it is purely muscular trouble you have got at the moment, there is no joint trouble at all. Okay? 'Bye-bye.'"

Both in a medical sense and a psychological sense it is difficult to fault this consultation. The doctor has asked all the right questions, coped with the problems presented by the patient in medical and social terms and left the patient with some understanding of his condition. One might well suggest that his style here is perfectly suited to both the problem and the patient.

119

We now turn to look at Dr B—— attempting to cope with a very clearly presented problem of "depression". The patient needs little prompting to get her to talk about her condition so he is never faced with the problem of having to dig out his initial diagnosis. In this consultation observe how his questioning style is very similar to the style he showed in the previous consultation.

(Dr B—— .)

D. "Would you like to have a seat here Mrs Z——? You are a new patient aren't you? How long have you been in X—— town then?"

P. "Just a week."

D. "And you have brought this from your previous doctor?"

P. "I have."

D. "Yes, your doctor has written to say that after having a baby that four months after the baby you developed a depression, which he has been treating with some yellow pills for the last two months now. Otherwise things seem to be all right. Have you noticed any change in yourself since you took the yellow pills?"

P. "Not really."

D. "What is your chief complaint now?"

P. "Just depression, and just uninterested in anything really."

D. "Yes, all the things that you do as a married woman, the housework, looking after your husband, the sexual side of marriage, looking after the child. Which is the most difficult?"

P. "The sexual side I think."

D. "Has it always been a difficult thing or is it just recently?"

P. "No. Just recently. Just this last couple of months, I felt depressed and tired and I just couldn't be bothered to do anything. And it was just the thought of going to bed at night. . . ."

D. "The thought of going to bed at night?"

Here we see the doctor trying to use "reflective questions". As we subsequently learned, this was quite intuitive because this doctor claimed that he had never before thought of reflective questions and far less had he ever considered their value. Sadly, he loses the value of the patient's response because he proceeds to follow that with another suggestion.

P. "For the sexual side."

D. "Oh, I see. But, generally, you have lost interest in most things?"

P. "Most things, yes."

D. "How are you sleeping when you go to bed?"

P. "Quite well. Maybe not sound. Most nights I get a good rest, but I thought if I slept too much, would that have any effect as well?"

D. "I have never heard of people sleeping too much with a baby of three months or so. Can you explain what you mean?"

P. "Well, I usually go to bed about ten and up about eight. But one day I was up earlier and I thought I felt slightly better, at being up early in the morning."

D. "But on the whole you are sleeping well?"

P. "Yes."

D. "Do you enjoy your food?"

P. "Oh, yes."

D. "Is your weight steady?"

120

P. "Yes."

D. "When you say depressed can you explain what you mean by that? It means different things to different people."

He decided he was getting nowhere with his previous line of questioning and so he reverted to the very first problem offered. He did have an opening when she mentioned that one morning she felt better when she was out of bed very early. From then on, however, he spoiled his approach by asking closed questions which effectively stopped the patient from talking.

In the next set of interchanges he again repeats the same fault. Note how he is given an opening with the mention of "anger", which he virtually ruins because he tries to suggest to the patient what causes the anger. The fact that his relationship with his own child might make him angry is no basis for suggesting that the patient's child might be the cause of her anger. When this leads nowhere he tries to go back in time to examine her illnesses prior to her depression. That also leads nowhere and he then asks the question:

D. "What sort of things make you angry?"

P. "I feel that I could have a good cry at times. Nothing in particularly really, I could just have a good cry, and I feel that I would maybe be better."

D. "Are there certain things that make you feel that you want to cry?"

P. "No. I just get angry with myself. I want to do things but I just . . . and I get angry with myself."

D. "I see. How many children have you now?"

P. "Just the one."

D. "And do you feel that she is healthy enough?"

P. "Yes, I do. I think she is really quite happy apart from now, at night she is coughing, but I thought that might be with her teeth coming on."

D. "Before, when you went to your doctor, about feeling depressed, were your complaints any different then?"

P. "No. Just the same really."

D. "I see. And what sort of things make you angry?"

P. "Well, I feel that I would like to do something, dust or something like that. But with moving house I just don't have the energy to do anything like that and I just sit. And I feel after that I should have done it. And that is what makes me angry with myself. Just not going ahead and doing it."

D. "Yes. And before this, did you used to be an energetic person?"

P. "Quite energetic. I was a hairdresser, and I was never tired, well, not often. Not like this, and we were busy on our feet all day and I never felt this tired."

D. "I see. So how do you like being a housewife and mother?"

P. "I enjoy being a housewife and a mother."

D. "Say, for example, your husband comes home later than he should, how are you then?"

P. "Angry."

D. "And have you always been inclined to be angry? I mean after you got married and he came in later."

P. "Not really. . . ."

D. "Are there any other things that irritate you or make you angry? How does noise effect you, for example, the baby crying, or the TV on or the radio on?"

121

P. "I like the radio on. About the baby crying, well, I don't mind for a short time, but if she was to cry for quite a while, I feel I am getting tensed up. Otherwise, I don't think noise or anything does really affect me."

D. "Have you any funny fears or worries at the moment? You know, women are funny creatures . . . or fear that because they are not interested in sex that their husband will go elsewhere."

P. "Yes, I have."

D. "Fears of getting pregnant again, or making a fool of themselves. What fears have you got?"

P. "Well, the sexual side of it. Like fear of your husband going to someone else, or, most of these things you have said. Like making up the baby's feed, after you have done it, you wonder if you have done the right thing. Because your mind is just not set on it. On what you are doing."

D. "Yes. Can you explain, give an example of when this bothered you?"

P. "Well, just yesterday after I made up her feed, I thought have I done it or have I not and when I did look to see if I had made up her feed I wondered if I had done it properly."

D. "How many times did you go back and see if you had done the right thing, put the right number of scoops in the bottle?"

P. "Just the once."

D. "Do you ever get any other funny little fears, that you might have put something that will harm the baby in the bottle?"

P. "No. I have never feared of that, no."

D. "Do you often have to check things, for example at night that you have locked the doors, get up and check the doors?"

P. "I have, yes. Especially . . . I used to be the one that always locked the doors last thing, but now I just seem to forget. I just don't bother about things like that."

D. "How often do you get your husband to get up and check that the doors are locked?"

P. "Most nights, after I am in bed, I ask him if he has checked the doors. And he will sometimes say yes, and sometimes no, and he will have to get up again."

D. "So that is a change as well."

P. "Yes."

D. "What about other things, checking that the windows are open or closed, or that switches are off, or that the immersion heater is off?"

P. "No. I check that the heater is off. But I always did do that. I go upstairs and by the time I get there I have to stop and think what it was that I went up for."

D. "So your memory is a bit slippery at the moment?"

P. "Yes. I just don't seem to be able to concentrate."

D. "How near to the shops are you?"

P. "Well, I don't really know the shops yet, I don't know where things are. Every time I go I come home without things, even though it is written down."

D. "You could kick yourself when you get home."

P. "Yes."

D. "Tell me, have you ever felt this way before?"

122

P. "No."

D. "Can you remember any time when you were just the way you are now?"

P. "I can't say that I have, maybe for a day, have off days, but never for as long as this."

D. "Before you got married did you have any complaints like this?"

P. "No."

D. "While you were at school, before exams, did you ever feel tense or sweaty or . . .?"

P. "Well, I think I have always been a bit nervy, that sort of person. If there is anything exciting to be happening, I get nervous. But never so much as to bother."

D. "How were you during pregnancy?"

P. "I was sick all the time, and heartburn. The whole nine months."

D. "I see, yes. And when you knew you were pregnant, how did you feel about it?"

P. "Well, we weren't married at the time, well we were happy about it, but it was just a worry, but everything turned out okay. And we were glad to be getting married. We were going to get married anyway. I was depressed when I was pregnant, because of this sickness and heartburn, I feel that it has never really cleared."

D. "So you have been really unwell for quite a long time then?"

P. "Yes. I wouldn't say seriously ill, just this. . . ."

A psychiatrist who studied this consultation commented that the doctor suddenly unearthed an important part of the problem in a singularly unskilful fashion. Having done so he then lost his nerve and from this point on becomes desperately anxious to finish this consultation. The psychiatrist felt that at this point he would have started to probe for feelings of guilt stemming back to the early part of her pregnancy.

Whether one is prepared to accept psychiatric interpretation or not, it is apparent that the doctor does now start to accelerate the termination of the consultation. The doctor obviously has formed some sort of opinion but only offers oblique insights to the patient. From what he says it seems reasonable to suggest that he, too, suspected he was dealing with something stemming from the early part of the pregnancy.

Notice also the similarity in the two terminations. With the rheumatic patient the termination is full of fairly definite statements by the doctor. This consultation, with much less information to guide him, also ends on a fairly strong note.

D. "Yes, right. I think it will help you if you could talk about this at length, when you can take your time about it. Could you come at a special time and talk about this? You tell me that the pills are really not helping you and you have noticed no improvement. I think it would help you if you could talk about the feeling you had when you were pregnant. Could you do that?"

P. "Yes."

D. "Because at the moment you are in a normal surgery and we are always a little bit more busy then. So could you come up this Friday afternoon to talk about it?"

P. "Yes."

D. "So go to the desk and make a special appointment and they will give you an appointment for twenty to thirty minutes. Could you ask your husband to come with you? Would he be willing to come with you?"

P. "If he can get time off."

D. "Well, if he could get time off, I would like him to come and talk about you, not about himself. Okay?"

P. "Yes. Saturday afternoon is no good is it?"

D. "No, I am afraid not. Could you go down to the desk and make another appointment for Friday afternoon, and you can take your time about talking your fears, during pregnancy, because I am sure this has got a lot . . . a lot to do with why you are not feeling right."

P. "Yes, I really feel that. My last doctor, she asked what was wrong but never. . . ."

D. "Well, if you come back on Friday, you can take your time, particularly about how you felt when you fell pregnant. And also your feeling towards the baby during pregnancy. Okay. In the meantime I am not going to change the pills that you are already on. We will go into that when you come back on Friday. Okay?"

P. "I finished those tablets just yesterday."

D. "I see. Well, I will give you some other tablets just to help you temporarily, until we have gone into this. Because really, I am not convinced that you are depressed in the sense that you need to go to the mental hospital. You are not depressed in that sense."

P. "I worry about that, you know."

D. "You are not as bad as that."

P. "I don't think that I am but I wonder if it will come to that."

D. "I don't think so. No. It won't come to that. And in the meantime you take these, one twice a day and two in the evening. Okay? So make an appointment for Friday afternoon. ' Bye-bye."

Looking at the consultations we have quoted in this chapter and those we quoted in Chapter 9, one conclusion seems to suggest itself time and again. When a doctor develops his style there is a possibility that it can be a sort of prison within which the doctor will be forced to work. In the last consultation it was evident that the doctor was trying hard to get some sort of leads from the patient but did not seem to have the basic skills. He was also unable to stop himself suggesting even when he was wrong two out of three times. In the training programme we referred to earlier, this doctor decided to learn the skills of "reflecting", "seeking patient ideas" and "using patient ideas". He admitted at the time that these were totally new concepts to him. If one accepts the idea that "reflecting" is a behaviour pattern, it must also be accepted that new behaviours are difficult to learn unless one has a clear idea of what the behaviour might be.

Given the fact that doctors work in isolation of each other and are thus without any agency which can offer feedback on their performance it is difficult to see how they can change their styles. A doctor has to know what "reflecting" is before he can use it as a conscious strategy. Furthermore, he needs to know how to use all the other skills which accompany "reflecting" to make it an effective strategy.

There are a number of doctors who can and do adjust their styles. In conversation with these doctors one important factor has been agreed upon as a major determinant of style. The existence of a physiological crisis appears to force a doctor to act with little concern for his patient's feelings. Medical needs are paramount and the doctor is obliged to act as the sole agent. As one doctor put it: "A patient in the throes of a coronary thrombosis hardly needs a few well chosen questions about the intricacies of his sex life." Such a situation requires a strong doctor-centred approach. The problem is that the doctor-centred style is extremely seductive. As long as illness can be rationalised into standardised packages and as long as patients can be taught to produce standardised symptoms, then doctor-centred styles are good styles for doctors to use.

Another significant factor is the doctor's definition of what constitutes a "medical problem". The following consultation with a very distressed patient was considered by seven other GPs. Five of them declared that this patient should not have been allowed to continue for more than two minutes and that her problems were not the concern of a family doctor. They suggested all sorts of other agencies which might have been concerned but were adamant that this patient should not be a medical problem. They considered that psychiatric hospitals, priests, social workers or even prisons could cope with this set of problems more effectively.

In this case the patient found a sympathetic doctor who, in his own words, "had not the faintest idea what to do with her at the time but felt if she were kept talking something might emerge". His personal view was that this patient did fall within his orbit of concern even though he was not equipped to cope with her. It is doubtful if anyone could have helped this patient at the time of the reported consultation, but the doctor concerned felt that over a long period he could do something to help her.

Judging by the responses of other doctors to this patient's consultation one concludes that whilst she is of a type not completely strange to many doctors, they would prefer such patients to go elsewhere with their problems. They define medicine in a rather more narrow organic fashion than this reported particular doctor and would have shifted responsibility for her elsewhere with rapidity.

Dr C——.

D. "Come in. What sort of week-end have you had?"

P. (Unable to hear patient clearly.) "Ten years today, ten. Six seemed fairly all right. . . . But shattered on Friday, cried and cried. I baby-sat for my next-door neighbour. Saturday he . . . yesterday, that's when it took place." (Patient mumbles, unable to hear clearly.)

D. "What are you going to do without them?"

P. "I don't know. That's it, that's the end, that's the finish."

D. "What do you mean, that's the finish?"

P. "I am just not taking another bloody. . . . They took me into hospital and they pumped me full of muck, and this is the result. Fifteen years . . . your baby . . . they could have helped my child. You know that, don't you, admit it to me. This and all the other muck I. . . . (Patient whispers inaudibly for 15 seconds.)

P. "I'm panic-stricken, he's bloody mad, his brother. . . . Dr C—— I arrived here to find a woman, running away from three children, sitting in the park at night. I didn't know what was going on. I just thought . . . she must be mad, there must be something wrong with her. Now I look back . . . who should have been in that hospital, me or him, that girl's parents were as sane, if not saner than mine. Salt of the earth, English. And I have not just given in, I have tried seven bloody times to kill myself. Not because I wanted to die, because I thought it would be a blessed release for the likes of them. Well, all right, he has had his blessed release. All right, you don't commit adultery, you don't have babies and you don't be an illegitimate parent. And you don't have a lover. But I had mine . . . nothing except humiliation and insults. Today he's. . . . I didn't ask for it. Three times in this past year . . . if you saw the letter I wrote to him last week, and the phone call to help me. You would have said, why didn't you ask me how to. . . . You would have said it. It's his children's birthday this month, at Christmas time I was short, because of that, I can't be short with. . . . I am living now on my nerves . . . I walk the floor. . . . They wonder why I am in and out . . . am I to look forward to the rest of my life in that place. This woman. . . . 'Just a short note. . . . I have been trying to find possible jobs for you.' I don't want a possible job, I should have had my child. They help other people. Dr C——, either I am mad, ill or just a write off. If that is the case then why am I not in hospital? Why has S—— admitted defeat? Dr C——, you are a man, you are my age, perhaps a little older, do you know what I am talking about?"

D. "Yes, I do."

P. "Do you know what those children meant to me?"

D. "Yes."

P. "Do you know what that man meant to me?"

(Unable to hear patient.)

P. ". . . such a man, he took our lives . . . and he threw them into the gutter. . . . This . . . lady comes to see me, Mrs A——, and I couldn't talk to her. . . . I spent my time apologising, begging and scraping the bloody floors. I am not made that way. Do you understand, I am not mad, I grew up with a woman like your wife, I walked the same with my mother as your wife walks with her children. . . . But what she does is no mystery to me. I can appreciate it because that is how I grew up. And that is how . . . should have grown up with me. I couldn't help . . . my baby. They brought her to me . . . deplorable, you will admit, revolting circumstances. . . . I tried to kill myself. . . . Dr C——, they brought her to me and they said find accommodation. . . . You know J——, she came to me and said, she is not the only one, there was one in hospital. . . . My job is with my child, I've signed the paper, to give her away, gave my flesh and blood away. There are three children next door, your children, I have not even seen them. . . . I am no stranger to children because I love them. . . . You can't pretend with children, can you?"

D. "No."

P. "Can you? Do I speak sanely or insanely? Do I make sense?"

D. "Yes."

P. "You cannot lie to children. You might be able to pull the wool over their eyes when they are one month old but after that it is very difficult. Her little three-year-old wants to share her bed with me. She hardly knows me. . . . I don't go there much because they are a family and I won't impose on

126

them . . . that could be my child. I should be walking with my child . . . why could they not help me? What do they think these will do, cure the heartache and the heartbreak?"

D. "No. How can they?"

P. "What do they think sitting in a bed-sitter or behind a typewriter. All right, I worked as a young girl . . . but some of us are born just to be cabbages, as the saying goes, these days. . . . I want my children."

D. "How often do you see . . . these days?"

P. ". . . with her boy-friend. The sister . . . lives next door to my husband, who I wouldn't even wipe the gutter with. . . . That is what my children have come to. . . . I nearly died with all three of them you know. Bring me my baby . . . under those circumstances . . . put your heads together and you got me the hell out of there. Which was, I suppose, something to be thankful for . . . bed-sitter, I once had a home, I have always put a roof over our heads. I kept the roof over our heads on what he had I kept the roof . . . having to repay and he turns round today and tells me I haven't got any friends . . . all right it takes two wrongs to make a right, whichever way you look at it . . . when I arrived in England to see another woman, a woman I didn't know, with three children. This particular bitch must stay out of my life, I once threatened, that if I see her I will do her physical damage. He is the legal father of. . . . If I hadn't signed that, he could have signed it over and above my head, do you know that? So I signed, not because I wanted to but because I wasn't going to give him the last say in the matter. I want to show you something. Just pretend they are dead, I told you that's what she said to me once. How can I ever pretend? Could you, could you?"

D. "Can you?"

P. "No. Is that so difficult to understand?"

D. "I understand it. Do sit down."

P. "This I was going to tear up. I am not going to tear it up because I am not happy about the fact that there are . . . doctors. And I never shall be. Because they could have helped me with my . . . as they helped others. A helpless girl off the road, who got drunk on the strength of a bottle of bloody cheap wine. I wanted that child. . . . I returned her. On the strength of . . . gullible . . . (reading from letter) '. . . the position of . . . which he accepted and treated as part of the family'. He never accepted her, he might have treated her, he treated her, well as he put it to me he wouldn't throw a sick woman out and he wouldn't ill-treat a baby. But as a child of the family, nonsense. 'Has frequently taunted.' I never said a word. He kept on and on about J——. I said, do you want him to knock at your door. I told him he wasn't a man's backside, and he is not."

(Confused noise.)

P. (Reading from letter.) " 'Has frequently used vulgar, abusive language, and has on occasions done so in front of the children.' There is no mention of him knocking me around. And using language on me, and treating me like a whore. How does he explain away? That those children looked forward to the baby. They wanted the baby. They used to ask me, 'Mummy, why don't we have a baby? Our baby.' "

(Confused noise.)

127

P. "This is the decree nisi, incidentally. 'Provided that if either parent do not give a general undertaking to return the said child. . . .' Now make up their minds, am I or am I not in a fit state to care for my child?"

D. "Can I tell you that?"

P. "I asked you . . . have your baby adopted. Why didn't you people put your heads together and say, 'Look, this woman needs her child. Let us help her.'"

D. "The child has to have an income though, and a roof and somebody who's able to look after her."

P. "But why am I unable to care for my child?"

D. "Well, why?"

P. "Oh, come on then, tell me why."

D. "Can you go out to work?"

P. "I could care for my child, if I had been given the help, and wasn't subjected to these things. Which I needn't have been to start with. That's all I am, a bloody drug addict. I wasn't asking or making. I am not going to see J—— and I am not going to see G——."

D. "What are you going to do then?"

P. "I don't know . . . don't bloody care. It doesn't make any difference any more. I don't know what to do about this. . . . l have got to pay this week's rent. I could have cared for M——. . . . They helped J——, she came to me in tears, M——, what shall I do? I said, 'If you want your child . . . back to your parents.' So she stood up to them and she has got P——. All right, they have lost their shop, so what? What is a shop to a child? If it was your practice and your children at stake, what would you choose?"

D. "My children."

P. "Right. But I have had no choice, I have been stuck with those things, others worse, why? Because of a man who took it upon himself to throw our lives into the gutter. And I was carted off to hospital and now my daughter spends her time with a . . . grotty grovelling snob. Miserable, wretched lot of yobs. Likely to fall pregnant at seventeen, she is now."

D. "I know."

P. "And! Now he paints the doors and the ceiling."

(Confused noise.)

P. "There was a girl in that hospital, C—— by name. Chopping herself up with razor-blades and little bits of, you name it, but they helped her. . . ."

The consultation lasted another two or three minutes and the patient left with a prescription and another appointment scheduled for the following week. Medically, it is fair to comment that the doctor has done very little. One must also add that his patience is quite monumental. From our point of view the consultation is important because it represents a type of problem which most GPs would be unwilling to, or incapable of, handling. The doctor has allowed the patient to talk and talk in the belief that such talking is in itself therapeutic. All the doctor has done is to make encouraging noises and listen. He has also given up 17 minutes of his time.

Doctors also make judgements about the ability of a patient to understand medical problems, and about the ability of a patient to become involved in the management of his own condition. Some of the doctors researched in this work have given very clear-cut answers to this question.

128

"Treat patients like you treat drivers in front and behind—always expect them to do something stupid."

"I see no reason at all to explain a patient's condition to him. If he asks an intelligent question I might offer some simple explanation—but on the whole I prefer not to."

"How can you expect a layman to understand the sort of language we talk. Very few of my patients would have the faintest idea what was wrong with them even if I were to explain it to them."

The doctor who considered patients to be similar to motorists provided a series of consultations in which he demonstrated a remarkable ability to see a patient every three minutes. In this example we see him dealing with a patient at the end of a normal busy surgery. It should be added that the doctor dislikes this patient because he is a persistent drunk. It was pointed out by a lecturer in a medical school that the patient did intimate that he was prepared to learn something with his question about the meaning of "side-effects". The doctor refused the opportunity to educate his patient.

D. "Good morning. What is it then?"

P. "I've got some sort of inflammation here. I'm not sure what caused it but it's not too comfortable."

D. "Yes. Let's have a look. Mmm. Mmm."

P. "Do you think it could be caused by those tablets I started last week?"

D. "No. Turn round, let's have a look at the back of the leg. Mmm. Mmm."

P. "Well, it all started twenty-four hours after I changed tablets."

D. "Those tablets have no side-effects."

P. "What's side-effects?"

D. "Never mind. Can you walk comfortably?"

P. "Yes. I can't wear those heavy winter underpants though. Do you think it's caused by wool or something like that?"

D. "No."

P. "I got soaked last week. I fell into a gutter and had to walk home all dripping wet. Is that it?"

D. "Maybe. Right, take this to Mr. C——. Rub it on until it's gone."

P. "You'll see when he makes it up. 'Bye-bye."

Despite the doctor's antipathy it does seem that doctor and patient are satisfied with their respective roles.

One of the phenomena we investigated concerned the curious fantasies doctors develop about appointment systems. It was observed that a number of doctors held consultations which became progressively shorter as the surgery wore on. At first it was assumed that this was caused by tiredness or a need to leave the surgery at a particular time. Six of the doctors concerned in these observations were asked to explain this phenomenon and all hotly denied that they had such a variation because all claimed to run rigid appointment systems.

At present the evidence of this research is that doctors who establish appointment systems run the danger of establishing a dichotomy of objectives. Each doctor organises his appointment system around his perception of what constitutes the average time for a patient to pass through his surgery. When a particular patient uses up more than his allotted time (from our tapes, a probability of one in ten) then the doctor is trapped between:

(a) his desire to maintain good management over the actual patient in the consulting-room;

(b) his desire to manage his time in such a way that he keeps his appointment with the next patient in the waiting-room.

The six doctors volunteered information about their time-scheduling arrangements. As a non-random group of six they are too small and too badly selected to be a good sample but the information they provided is remarkably consistent. All worked to a five or six minute schedule, but had never kept any records to demonstrate how quickly they actually turned over patients. All took between 30 to 90 seconds longer to consult each patient than their predicted time for the first two-thirds of a surgery. Thus, they would spend between five-and-a-half and seven minutes. Then in the last one-third of the surgery they compensated by holding consultations which last from two-and-a-half to three minutes. They all claimed that the shortening was quite unconscious, but did admit that they were aware of severe time-pressure at the end of most surgeries.

The late Dr Burns of Salford volunteered some data he collected from 11 doctors in the Greater Manchester area. He discovered a fantasy which covered most of his 11 doctors. These doctors ran morning surgeries based upon a notional six minutes per patient. The surgery itself ran for two-and-a-half hours but patients were only scheduled in three half-hour periods within that two-and-a-half hours, ie, five patients in 30 minutes. The doctors claimed that the remaining hour was made up of two rest periods of 30 minutes each. Burns noted that not one of these doctors could remember a time in the previous three weeks when they had taken a 10 minute rest period let alone 30. The doctors were, in fact, permitting their patients to fill up the resting time. Burns claimed to have confronted these doctors with the idea that they deliberately worked their schedules in this way because they knew they could not cope with more than seven or eight patients per hour.

We have observed earlier that some doctors do alter their styles slightly when dealing with patients of the opposite sex or even with children. One final observation is that there are a number of doctors who change their style of terminating a consultation quite markedly when dealing with an old-age pensioner. Here is a typical example of the way in which one particular doctor terminates his consultations:

D. "Okay. Now then. It's not very serious but there are a few things I want you to do. Firstly, I want you to go to the hospital and have that arm X-rayed. Now then, I don't want you to start worrying but I can't see inside there and I want to be quite sure that nothing is badly broken."

P. "Well, the pain does keep me awake in the night."

D. "Yes, yes, I'm sure it does. It must be very painful if it keeps you awake. I think you ought to have come in last week when you fell off that bike. Still, I'll tell you what, I'll give you a few tablets to get you to sleep. Now then, these tablets are marvellous. They are quite safe and even if in mistake you swallow the lot you will only sleep longer. Take one in the night and if you wake up too early then maybe you can take another."

P. "I'm not too keen on tablets."

D. "No, and quite right too. We eat far too many tablets you know. These are quite safe. I only prescribe these now you know. You see, you'll sleep like a top. Now then, I'll fix for you to go up to the hospital and get that X-ray. M—— will give you a ring. Okay? We've got your number. There it is. Good, okay. Right, see you soon. 'Bye-bye."

There is something of the mother-hen clucking over her brood in this approach. In the same tape there are three interviews with old-age pensioners. These all receive the same detailed examination, but the closures are quite different and start when he returns to his chair having conducted a physical examination:

Closure 1

"More of the same S——. Right-ho. Take this off to the chemist. Three times a day after meals. Same as before. Okay? Ta-ta now."

Closure 2

"Legs still stiff, then? Right-ho. Well now, keep the dressings up. There's a note for some more. Okay? Pick it up tonight. Save a trip, eh? Ta-ta now."

Closure 3

"Well, there's nothing wrong with her, Mr W——. Don't worry about it. No, she'll be okay. Take this to the chemist. Okay? After meals. Ta-ta then."

Quite the reverse behaviour has been observed with another GP who spent at least three times his normal amount of time when dealing with old-age pensioners. He is quite unable to account for this curiosity although he is very much aware of it.

Our evidence leads us to conclude that the majority of GPs seem to evolve, largely by trial and error, a relatively static style of consulting. This style, however, may be influenced by the following factors:

(a) the degree of crisis perceived by the doctor;
(b) the sex of the patient;
(c) the age of the patient;
(d) the degree of pressure created by overrunning time schedules.

We have not been able to discover any real evidence to suggest that the following factors seem to influence a style:

(a) the social class of the patient;
(b) the verbal skills of the patient;
(c) the degree to which the problem is non-organic in origin.

NB. With reference to the social class of patients we must admit that our evidence is incomplete. The majority of practices involved in this study were urban practices and, as such, tended to serve the needs of immediate localities. As such we have been unable to compare a large number of doctors interacting with patients drawn from a wide spectrum of social class backgrounds. The consultations we have studied reflect the social class range covered by the practice, and in the majority of cases this does tend to be very narrow.

CHAPTER 12
UTILISING THE RESEARCH

So far we have concerned ourselves with the information produced by the first phase of our study. We conclude that we can, with tape recordings of 20 consecutive consultations, predict more than 80 per cent of a doctor's behaviour pattern. We can also establish his preferred styles of relating to patients for diagnosis and for prescription. This information might be interesting as the subject of an esoteric PhD, but as such it is of no practical value. The next three chapters of this book are concerned with our various attempts to turn our information into a training tool.

The first and most obvious use we have found is the value of the audio tape recording. We have already written about this in *Learning to Care* (second edition, 1975). Simply listening to tape recordings of one's own performance is, at times, traumatic but often instructive.

The task we have set ourselves is to provide a set of instruments with which the solo learner may provide himself with feedback to facilitate his self-learning. The obvious instrument we have so far provided is the behavioural interpretation of an interview. We suggested that six stages or phases might be observed:

    I Greeting and relating
    II Discovering the reasons for attendance
    III Conducting a verbal or physical examination or both
    IV A consideration of the condition
    V Detailing further treatment
    VI Terminating the interview.

Taking three short sample consultations from one of our tapes we can examine them to see how they measure against this simple check list. As each of the phases occurs it will be denoted by the appropriate Roman numeral.

Example 1 is one of a series of consultations between this doctor and this particular patient, and every Tuesday this patient returns for further on-going treatment. For the previous seven visits the patient has been content to go away with his prescription, but now the doctor is in the process of trying to wean the patient off one drug, which has a habituating risk, on to another.

Example 1

D. (I) "Come in. Hello. (II) How are you?"

P. "I feel shocking. You know, when I came to see you last week and you knocked those capsules off—well, every morning when I get up, and my head—Doctor you could have amputated it. It was a terrible headache and it was as if somebody was dragging my eyeballs out. So I took more tablets, I haven't had anything since . . . swollen, I've had bags under my eyes and all snuffly and watery, and at the moment, all the top of my head here feels as though there's pressure on it and I feel this stuff going down the back of my throat."

D. (III) "Are you coughing any of it out?"

P. "No, I can't cough it out as . . . when I blow my nose it's clear."

D. "Is your nose blocked? Lie your head back and I'll have a look."

P. "Just here and inside of my throat is always very tender and all under here , . . and with both my hands tucked underneath my ribs and my head feels as if it's going to fall off."

D. (V) "Well, I'll give you a change of tablets for that and when you're over this I'll start you back on the capsules."

P. "Well, all the aches and pains have gone, apart from under my ribs."

132

D. (VI) "Well, leave it a week and come and see me again. (IV) It sounds as if it's the cold that's affecting your sinuses. (VI) Right, so a week from today."

P. " 'Bye-bye, now."

The sequence in this consultation is I–II–III–V–VI–IV–VI.

When we examined other consultations volunteered by this doctor we found that Phase IV is one which he rarely used. In a discussion of the above consultation he was asked to explain why he had given the piece of information:

"It sounds as if it's been the cold that's affecting your sinuses."

His explanation was fascinating:

"I was very angry that my attempt to get her off that stuff wasn't working. She had not followed her instructions and had taken too many at once and then suffered for a week. I should have given her a right piece of my mind. Instead I decided not to upset her and to get her out as soon as possible. I thought I had got rid of her with the 'come and see me again' but she just sat. It was really meant to reassure her so that she would go away. In fact, it was a useless consultation because we were both running away from the reality of her condition. Unless there's a miracle she's only got a few months. I have not told her but I'm sure she knows."

In fact, his speed in this consultation, especially his short Phase II, are indicative of a much greater problem he had with this patient. Whilst all six stages were present at least two were misused.

His next consultation was with a patient returning after referral to a hospital. This patient had a long history of back trouble which reached a crisis some four weeks previous to this interview. When the patient arrived the doctor had not the faintest idea why he was there, because the consultation following the referral was not due to take place for another week. As soon as the patient refers to his consultation with the specialist the doctor remembers a letter which arrived that morning—hence the conversation with the receptionist. He has not yet had time to assimilate the specialist opinion, and throughout the whole interview he admits to not having had the faintest idea why the patient was there.

Example 2

D. (I) "Hello. Come and sit down Mr T——. (II) How are you?"

P. "Well, they've managed to get things rushed through from . . . and they brought it forward and a fortnight ago I saw Dr G—— and he said it was disc trouble of long-standing and he asked me if I've ever had an accident, well, you see, I've had several, but many years ago."

(Two-minute pause—conversation with receptionist.)

D. "Yes, many years ago. (IV) Well, I've had a letter from him and he says the reversing the lorry doesn't help much, with your having to turn your head. . . ."

P. "Well, that's what I'm a bit worried about you see."

D. "He's given you a collar, but that's only for the night isn't it? (III) He's putting you on the physiotherapy?"

P. "Yes. I went yesterday."

D. (V) "It's a bit early yet to see if you're going to have any effect from it."

P. "Aye. About three weeks yet."

133

D. (III) "What is your job?"

P. ". . . Well, I'm on a quarry job, carting clay, as a slagger—it's a very rough job—that's the trouble . . . well, I've been seriously thinking about getting a lighter job if I could and I'm travelling to Denton but it would be out on the moors type of thing."

D. (V) "Oh, well, that's no good to you . . . and this business of turning your head round most of the time, you see you're putting a strain on your neck."

P. "I have to move back into the yards."

D. "Oh, that's no good to you. It's enough trouble if you've got your neck normal. It would be better if you could find a job—this is a fairly new job, isn't it? Were you on long distance before that?"

P. "Well, I was on middle distance actually, it wasn't as strenuous."

D. "It might be better to look for something lighter. (III) How old are you now?"

P. "Fifty-three."

D. (V) "It's not the time of life to start looking for another job, is it? I was thinking of a light van or something of that sort."

P. "Aye, that's right."

D. "In the meantime, though, do you find you can manage your job or do you want to give it a week's rest?"

P. "Give it a week's rest. It's a bit awkward. I've got three weeks to go and I'm going up to Denton and keeping nice and warm and I'm going up there and going against it really."

D. "I think you'll have a better chance of improving it. . . ."

P. "If I'm off?"

D. "Yes, I think so. The X-rays show quite a lot of damage in the joints."

P. "While I've been on that job I've been really bad at times, you know. . . ."

D. "Have they given you any tablets?"

P. "Well, I've got those tablets you gave me."

D. "Have you many left?"

P. "Yes, quite a few yet."

D. "I'll give you a note for a week—and has he provided you with this collar? You've got the collar?"*

P. "Yes. For the night time, you know."

D. "During the day keep your neck well wrapped up. Try not to turn it more than you have to. Keep it warm. At the hospital you're having—heat—oh, you're not having exercise, yet, oh, just the heat. Try not to use your neck more than you have to. When you think you're ready then they will show you some exercises then you can do those. In the meantime, I would advise you to look around for something a bit more suitable, while you're off. You see, this is permanent damage. They will get you a lot of relief with the treatment but you will always be liable to more trouble. If you stayed in the same job you would most likely stir it up again. . . . (Pause.) (VI) Anyhow, give it a week and let me have a look at you again. 'Bye-bye now. Good night."

An analysis of the structure of this consultation reveals some of the mess the doctor is in:

I–II–IV–III–V–III–V–III–V–VI.

134

He is clearly having to revert to Phase III as a method of keeping control over what he was doing. This might well be a charitable interpretation as the asterisk indicates another area in which the doctor might well be indulging in yet some more Phase II behaviour. As he already has this information it seems redundant.

This, as the doctor admitted, was the result of not being quite ready for the events of the day. What he claimed to have found interesting was his inability to hold the events whilst he took real stock of his situation. In retrospect, he felt that he should have read his own notes after the receptionist had given him the contents of the letter. He also admitted that he had strong feelings about the need to appear to be in control of events. Certainly, however, we learn from this that a continuing oscillation from III to V is indicative of some degree of confusion.

His last consultation that morning (below) he claims as his worst that day. This one concerns another ageing patient who appeared at the tail end of the morning surgery, after 23 others. The doctor by now was tired and knew that he had a considerable list of domiciliary visits.

Example 3

D. (I) "Hello. Come in. (II) How are you?"

P. "Got a cold. . . ."

D. (III) "It's the fashion this week, everybody's got it. Well now, how's the breathing going, any different?"

P. "Not so bad, doctor, can't grumble, I feel a bit better than I did before."

D. "That's a good sign. Are you coughing at all?"

P. "A bit, just got a bad chest, just my arms, you know."

D. (IV) "It's the cold and damp—that sort of thing. You didn't have another appointment, did you?"

P. "Oh, on Friday I had a letter from him saying that they've altered my appointment—they've altered it and brought it forward. . . ."

D. (V) "They've brought it from the fifteenth of March to the thirteenth of March. (IV) That's a funny postponement isn't it, unless they've reorganised the clinic. Dr Walker's away, anyway, anyway . . . probably a misprint. . . . (V) Are you taking those tablets, one in a morning, one heart tablet, three of . . . two of the other one and a spoonful of medicine, yes, well, I would like you to carry on with those, unless Doctor Walker wants you to change. Well, that's the fifteenth. I'll see you again before you go to the out-patients there, and we'll see how things are going."

P. "Will you see me before . . .?"

D. (VI) "Well, you're going on the thirteenth. That's the same day, isn't it? That's also on Tuesday, four weeks today. Well, if you make an appointment for say the Thursday, the fifteenth, tell me what he has to say, that will be better . . . he didn't mention in his letter, but very often he just forgets and lets the secretary sort it out. 'Bye-bye. . . ."

The sequence is as follows:

I–II–III–IV–V–IV–V–VI.

It will be noted that the VI has been placed at the start of his final set of statements. He is shutting the patient off completely by totally ignoring her request:

"Will you see me before . . .?"

135

(The case caused a subsequent difference of opinion with his partner. It transpired that the old lady was quite terrified about her referral and had probably come that morning to talk about it. The doctor had no idea at all why she was there and never gave her a chance to tell him. After the above consultation the patient requested a meeting with the partner, as it happened on an evening when her own doctor was not available. The partner got involved and decided to take his colleague to task about not caring for his older patients. The doctor concerned protested his innocence loudly and offered his recording as evidence. As may be observed, his "evidence" was more part of the case for the prosecution than for the defence.)

From this particular case the doctor claimed he learned to spend more time trying to be certain that he knew why the patient was there. His deficiency in Phase IV, however, left him unmoved, and subsequent recordings of his consultations indicate that he does try harder to find out why patients come but spends no more time discussing collected information with them.

There are, at times, considerable problems in knowing just what is happening in a consultation. Take the following case:

D. "Good morning, come in. Mrs L——, isn't it?"
P. "Yes."
D. "Now then, you have moved to Rochdale, haven't you?"
P. "Yes. I moved yesterday but I'm back."
D. "Back?"
P. "I don't like the house there."
D. "Where are you living now?"
P. "Where I were before."
D. "Oh, I see. Now then, what can I do for you?"
P. "Well, that's why I'm here."
Long silence.
D. "Yes?"
P. "Well, I'm here. I'm not at all well."
D. "Yes?"
P. "Well, you know."
D. "What?"
P. "Well, they said I should come and see you about the pill."
D. "Oh, the pill. Is that what you want?"
P. "Well, can I have it?"
D. "Well, yes. Have we spoken about this before? No, there's nothing here on your card. Let's see, how old are you? Thirty-seven. How many child. . . . You have no children. Why do you want the pill? What are you doing at the moment?"
P. "It's not for me, it's for her."
D. "Who?"
P. "Mrs D——."
D. "Mrs D——?"
P. "Aye, she lives next door."
D. "But I don't think she is my patient."
P. "Oh. Well, then I'll have my tablets then."
D. "Tablets?"
P. "Yes, you know, them blue ones."

136

D. "Oh, yes. Of course. Let's see. Ah, yes. You should have come in last week, shouldn't you. Mmm. There you are then. Take that off to the chemist."

P. "Can I show you this?"

D. "Good God! Where did you get that?"

P. "He done it last night. When I walked out."

D. "How long has it been bleeding?"

P. "Since last night."

D. "Right. Let's get it cleaned up."

P. "You'll not tell the cops, will you?"

D. "Tell the police? Why?"

P. "Well, I thought you had to every time you see something like this."

D. "For severe cuts and lacerations. Well, no."

P. "Oh, that's good. He hit me with a sheet of glass."

D. "A sheet of glass?"

P. "Aye, he threw it as I were leaving."

D. "Now, look, you are going to have to get this properly stitched. I think I had better send you up to the hospital. I'll get someone to run you up now and I'll phone them."

This is one of the few cases we have where the patient goes through such a complex set of manoeuvres before coming to the point. The doctor confessed to total and utter confusion right through until he saw the wound. He even admitted that he prescribed some more anti-depressant and skirted around the fact that she had been in the previous week. He hoped at that stage to get her out.

It is very difficult to know what a doctor should do in a case like this. Clearly there was something totally wrong with what the patient was saying, but there was no indication anywhere that the patient was more concerned about whether or not this doctor would call in the police because of a severe wound. Presumably the logical approach to personal confusion is to say something like:

"I have not the faintest idea why you are here, I do not understand what you are trying to tell me. Would you like to start again and tell me please what you are here for?"

It is sadly true to comment that this approach may well result in the patient leaving without any more being said.

Another area where attention can profitably be paid is in the area of prescribing—Phase V. Many doctors offer opinions which are splendid examples of how little they know about their patients. Take the following pieces of advice given to patients from social class E:

"You will have to find a different job. You are too old for labouring. Why do you not drive a van or something?"

"Don't you think you ought to retire? You must be near seventy now."

"Don't you think that you ought to find a job? I mean, you've been out of work for three weeks now."

or the following advice to an old-age pensioner:

"Sure you can afford the train fare to go there. I mean, it's not more than fifty pence. That's not a lot of money."

In all of these examples the doctors were, without doubt, well intentioned. What they lack is an understanding of the lives of their patients. Information like this suggests certain questions to ask of doctors. To what extent, for example, do doctors make sure that what they are saying to a patient is either relevant to that patient or even understood? Having made a decision about the condition of the patient and having made up one's mind about what to do it can be very seductive to do this:

"Right you are. Now then, take this along to the chemist. Take the tablets three times a day after meals. Take the medicine every night before you go to bed. You are not to take the medicine in the morning."

This particular piece of advice was given to a night shift worker who only ate two meals per day and went to bed in the morning. As a form of words, however, it is perhaps one of the most common forms of termination. Equally, one might well ask some doctors about the complexity of the instructions they offer patients. Take the following:

"Now then, the two-coloured tablets are to be taken three times daily. It doesn't matter whether you take them before or after meals but there should be an interval of about six hours between each one at a time. Then the yellow ones are to be taken in twos once a day. Then you have these purple ones which you already have, those you may take when you feel you need one. I would advise you to take them in the morning and in the evening and only one at a time. Okay? Have you got that? Good. 'Bye-bye."

Given that verbal messages are prone to some misinterpretation, it is worth wondering how much of the above advice the patient actually could remember.

There are other general considerations in the ending of consultations which can be considered. For example, when a doctor finds that he continually finishes consultations in the above fashion he should be asking himself whether or not this is the best way with all patients.

The other area which is often revealed in this sort of analysis is the "missed lead". Balint accurately described the sort of relationship imposed upon patients by some doctors in "The apostolic function" (see Balint, *The Doctor, His Patient and the Illness*). Very often patients will, however, make oblique offers of information during consultations or, worse, will make the offer in the form of a "by the way, doctor" just as the doctor thinks he has finished. In many of the consultations studied in this research there have been numerous occasions where quite clearly patients have been making oblique offers and doctors have been ignoring them. The "by the way" syndrome has been well documented in several places. Browne and Freeling have an excellent section on the subject. What is not well documented is the "concealed offer" made by patients. Let us look at a few examples.

D. "Come in. Sit down. Mr G——. Fine. Now then, what is it today?"
P. "Oh, nothing, doctor. I've just called for my prescription."
D. "Ah, yes. What do we have you on? Let me see."
P. "Aye. I always pick it up on Thursday."
D. "That's it. Ah, yes. Fifty milligrammes. Good."
P. "Yes, I always come on Thursday. You leave it with the girl on the desk."
D. "Everything all right then, is it?"
P. "Oh, no problem, really."
D. "How's Mrs G——? Is she getting about?"
P. "Well, she seems to be all right."
D. "You usually pick this up at the desk, don't you? Why have you come in today?"

138

This doctor had finally put two offers together and realised that something was being said to him. The consultation proceeded to discuss the patient's daughter who was causing her father quite severe problems.

The next example is of an offer missed. We join this consultation after the doctor has completed a physical examination, following on the "offer" of chest pain.

D. "Well, it seems to be okay. Nothing out of the ordinary there. Blood pressure perhaps a little high but not something we need worry about."

P. "That sounds good. Can I put my shirt on now?"

D. "Yes. Yes. Please do. I think you could perhaps tell me more about your diet. What was it you said you were eating now?"

P. "Well, I have lots of milk you know."

D. "Yes, but solids?"

P. "Well, I don't eat a lot of fat now, you know. You told me to leave them alone before, didn't you?"

D. "Well, yes. Are you getting the vegetables I spoke about?"

P. "I'm not eating those salads, you know. My wife gets cross when I refuse to eat some of the stuff she cooks."

D. "Okay. Are you eating fruit now?"

P. "Yes, I try to get a pound of apples every day. The wife doesn't like fruit, so I have to get it myself."

D. "Oh, well, that's not going to hurt, is it? Well now. Take this and get it made up. Come back in a week or so. See you then. 'Bye-bye."

When this was replayed to the doctor concerned he realised that the patient had not answered any question he had been asked. Moreover, he had made an offer about his wife which had been completely missed. This made the doctor angry because he already suspected that there were domestic problems which were interfering with his management of this case. He also offered some insight which was remarkably honest.

"I did not want to hear that sort of information at that time. If the bloody man had come in at the start of the surgery I would have got it 'in one'. At the end of a long surgery I'm just too tired to cope with that sort of information. As long as I am satisfied there is nothing life threatening I suspect that's what I'd do again."

Given the often excessive demands made upon the time of some GPs this sort of response probably reflects what many doctors feel about concealed offers from patients.

We have been able to define a number of phase sequences which might be described as "normal". Normality in this sense means that the consultation follows a sequence which appears to be logical, in that one set of events follows naturally upon another:

I–II–III–IV–V–VI is the sequence we have outlined in Chapter 3 and might well be the form taken by a complete new case.

I–II–III–V–VI is almost the same as above but omits the fourth phase, which we must admit can be seen as optional.

I–II–III–VI and

I–II–V–VI both describe a variety of situations, eg, on-going treatment or repeat prescriptions.

I–V–VI typical of many repeat prescriptions is more problematic. If there is no doubt at all as to the patient's reason for attendance then it might well be seen as "normal".

We have also been able to identify some consultation structures which may be regarded as being problematic, either for the doctor or for the patient. The most obvious is a structure such as the one below:

I–II III–V–III–V–III–V–VI.

One interpretation of what is happening in such a consultation is that the doctor is trying to close off the consultation before he is quite certain what he is doing. Alternatively, the reversion to Phase III may well be caused by the patient who is in a similar state of uncertainty and starts to volunteer more information which may serve only to confuse the doctor. The fact that the patient feels the need to do this ought to be significant to the doctor.

I–III–V–II–III–V–VI or
I–II–III–V–II–III–V–VI or
I–II–III–IV–II–III–V–VI

are all variations on the same theme. In every case the doctor is well advanced into his consultation when he discovers that the problem he thought he was dealing with is not the real patient problem. To the irritation of most doctors this realisation only occurs when they are well into the prescriptive part of a consultation.

A variation on the same theme is:

I–V–II–III–V–VI.

This is a common outcome of the doctor assuming that he is dealing with a repeat prescription and then discovering that the patient wants to talk about something new.

It is only fair to point out that many consultations will contain a quite natural reversion to an earlier phase, especially, for example, when the doctor is dealing with complex emotional problems. What is important is not that these "abnormal" patterns occur once, but that they occur with a frequency greater than three consultations in 10.

We have not selected three in 10 in a quite arbitrary manner. There is considerable debate between doctors about the number of emotional problems they are obliged to deal with in any given surgery. There is little disagreement that these problems constitute one of the most difficult areas of general practice. There is no agreement over what percentage of patients have emotional dimensions to the problems they bring to the doctor.

From the evidence we have it would seem that such problems can appear in consultations at the rate of about three in 10. The figure may well be an underestimate of the real incidence because some doctors are apt to stop patients before they have had the chance to say anything significant. What is clear, however, is that the rate of incidence is not less than three in 10, although they may be more common in a morning surgery than an evening surgery. There is also a slight positive correlation (0·56) between the incidence of female patients in a surgery and the apparent incidence of emotional problems.

After much discussion with doctors one has to accept that the training a doctor receives makes it unlikely that he will be able to cope easily with a non-organic problem. Whether those doctors who claim that they are only interested in organic problems are actually saying more than that they are incapable of coping with emotional problems must remain in doubt. What is

140

apparent is that few doctors seem happy when dealing with what one might describe as an "emotional offer".

It is very unlikely that the majority of doctors will be able to deal with a complicated and often concealed problem in the logical sequential pattern we have identified. Consequently, we would not describe as "abnormal" any such consultation which continually reverts to an earlier phase. To discover, however, that a doctor is reverting to previous phases at a rate greater than three in 10 consultations might well suggest that he is either trying to terminate the consultation too quickly or has not adequately discovered why the patient was there in the first place.

In order to use this information for the purposes of training both the trainer and the trainee should ideally have not just the tape recording but also a transcript of certain "key" consultations. The trainer would be concerned with a number of issues. A possible list of these might be as follows:

(a) The effectiveness of the trainee's attempts to discover why the patient is there (Phase II).

(b) The absence of any real Phase IV.

(c) The clarity of Phase V.

(d) The effects of deficient Phase II behaviour upon subsequent stages in the consultation.

(e) The incidence of reversion from a later phase to Phase II or III.

To conclude this chapter we offer readers an exercise in analysis. What must be discovered is how often the doctor reverts from Phase III to Phase II and how long he stays in this part of the consultation. There is no perfect answer, but various people have suggested that he changes from II to III or vice versa at least seven times (par is five). There are also two attempts at Phase IV.

D. "Come in. How are you?"

P. "I feel b—— all the time."

D. "Oh, dear. Can you tell me a bit more about it?"

P. "Well, I feel like I did before; my eyes feel proper heavy and my head. You know when I said before that I can't seem to keep myself awake."

D. "Yes."

P. "I feel like that."

D. "You're sleepy all the time?"

P. "Oh, no, I'm not sleeping all the time. I'm up early in the morning, every morning. I want to but I can't you know, but I'm half asleep all the time."

D. "You're half asleep?"

P. "I feel dopey, yeah."

D. "How do you sleep at night?"

P. "I were dreaming all last night but I don't usually, you know, I usually go off like a rocket."

D. "Yes, and what time do you waken up in the morning?"

P. "Well, he wakens me up."

D. "You wouldn't waken up apart from that?"

P. "No. I'd sleep on. Sometimes I don't hear him and our Carole has to get up and give me a shaking 'cos he stands up now and rattles the cot and shakes but I don't hear him half the time. Our Carole has to tell me and I have to get up."

D. "Yes. Do you feel the same all through the day?"
P. "I feel like that now, you know."
D. "How will you feel tonight?"
P. "I shall be dead tired, you know."
D. "You're just the same all through the day?"
P. "Yes."
D. "It doesn't get better?"
P. "Well, one day I can. . . ."
D. "I mean in one day. One day do you feel different or do you just feel like that all day?"
P. "Yes. I just feel tired all day. I have to make myself do my washing and. . . ."
D. "Can you concentrate?"
P. "What do you mean concentrate?"
D. "Well, if you have a little job to do, say you have to reckon up something in figures or say you want to read a book, would you not be able to do it because your mind wandered away from it?"
P. "No, I read, I read books, I'm always reading."
D. "You have no trouble reading books?"
P. "No, I've always read books. I like reading."
D. "How's your chest now?"
P. "Oh, it's all right."
D. "How do you feel about having an X-ray?"
P. "I don't know. I feel fed up, to tell you the truth. I never felt like this before I had him."
D. "Do you feel you've got something seriously wrong with you?"
P. "Sometimes I do, yes. Sometimes I frighten myself."
D. "Well, what do you think it is?"
P. "I don't know. Sometimes. . . ."
D. "An unknown thing?"
P. "Yes."
   Inaudible.
D. "How are things at home?"
P. "Oh, they're all right, you know."
D. "Does your mother help you?"
P. "Oh, yes."
D. "And your sister?"
P. "Very good. Oh, our Janet's married now, she's not at home. Our Carole's a good little soul, you know, she's very good with him."
D. "How old is Carole?"
P. "She's eleven. Yes, they're all very good, you know. No trouble there."
D. "Yes. Have you felt like going back to work?"
P. "Yes, I've felt like it but I'd be no use you know, working and coming home, I wouldn't be able to manage it, I know I wouldn't. No. (Inaudible.) I wouldn't be able to keep up with him. I mean if he's not well."
D. (Inaudible.) "I have this feeling at the back of my mind that you have a lot on and just thinking it out makes you tired. . . . What do you think about that?"
P. "I don't know. I don't think I am."
D. "How's your weight now?"

142

P. "I don't know, I've not weighed myself."

D. "Are you about the same, can you tell by your clothes whether you're gaining or losing?"

P. "I think I've lost a bit. I was nine stone, I don't know what I am now."

D. "Is there anything else you've not told me about?"

P. "No, not that I know of."

D. "Do you go out with your friends?"

P. "Oh, yes."

D. "You do. Would you like to have another opinion about it?"

P. "Yes."

D. "Well, I'll arrange for someone else to go over you and see if they can find anything wrong with you."

P. "Yes."

D. "Anyway, I'll tell you what I'll do. I'll write you out a letter and you can let Dr X see you at the hospital and tell him your story and see if he can tell you anything and we'll discuss it again afterwards. I'm going on holiday, but I'll see you again and we'll have a good talk about it."

P. "Yes."

D. "Okay then, if you tell the receptionist to make an appointment."

P. "When do you mean, this week?"

D. "Well, I'm going away tomorrow actually but I'll do it for you. You collect it tomorrow. Here you are then. All right? 'Bye-bye."

CHAPTER 13

ANALYSING DETAILED BEHAVIOUR AND DISCOVERING BASIC STYLES

This chapter deals with a use of the material which can only be achieved by using audio-tape recording. There is, as far as we can see, little to be gained in the analysis of verbal behaviour from visual examination of the consultation, so that a simple device such as an audio cassette recorder will be adequate.

Here we are concerned with the analysis of individual units of behaviour and how these may be scored on a prepared sheet.

It needs to be said that there is no such thing as the perfect style or the ideal set of behaviours. In the last resort doctors will use the styles which suit them best and which, in their terms, produce the sort of results they want. What we are concerned to say is rather more complex. There are some styles which will not work adequately with some combinations of patient and disorder. This needs clarification. There are some patients who prefer doctors to ask clear direct questions and who can give the doctor fairly clear and definitive responses in return. These patients will possibly behave in this fashion in consultations for most of the conditions which bring them into a surgery. Whether or not they would continue to do so if they themselves thought they were suffering from an illness which is socially frowned upon (eg syphilis) or from an illness of sinister import (eg cancer) is a debatable point.

We also have evidence that some styles are quite inadequate when dealing with non-organic illnesses. "Doctor centred"* styles seem to be inadequate when the doctor is faced with the patient who offers vague signs of emotional disorder yet few clear answers to direct questions. We must, however, indicate that it is not possible to offer absolute judgements on this last point. If a doctor does not intend to cope with vague symptoms, and if he fears that any sign of weakness on his part will encourage the patient to become a millstone around his neck, then he is likely to take refuge in a style which prevents emotion and feeling from entering into the consultation. Thus, when we say that "doctor centred" styles seem to be inadequate in most of those cases where patients finally present non-organic problems, we have to qualify that statement by accepting that many doctors intend to cope only with organic problems.

To avoid the need to make judgements concerning "good" and "bad" doctor behaviour, an effort was made to classify patient behaviour from the tapes in the same way that doctor behaviour had been classified. This exercise proved to be complex and confusing. The most significant evidence we have concerns four patients from the same practice who appear more than once in the collected tapes provided by the several doctors of that practice. On one of the visits made by each of these four patients they were seen by a doctor other than the one they normally consulted. In this context we refer to him as the "abnormal doctor". In each case the behaviour of the patient was totally different with the "abnormal doctor". Two of the patients were much more inhibited and less communicative, whilst the other two were much more communicative. Admittedly, on each occasion they presented different symptoms and thus may well have been suffering from quite different complaints—but none the less their behaviour was quite different from that exhibited to their usual doctor. What was stable in all of these consultations, however, was the pattern of behaviour produced by the doctor.

The two patients who became less communicative were "abnormally" consulted by a doctor who clearly exercises much more control over his patients than any other doctor in the practice. The two patients who became more communicative normally attended the "controlling" doctor referred to above, but were "abnormally" consulted by two doctors who are prepared to allow the patient to dictate a great deal of the pace of the consultation. While this particular evidence is interesting, subsequent discussions, in particular with Dr Paul Freeling and four other GPs in different practices in the north-west region, indicate that each was aware that such phenomena occurred within their own practices. It was, in fact, this abortive study of patient behaviour which produced the finding that in any series of consultations the behaviour of the doctor was singularly consistent whilst the behaviour of patients appeared to take a random pattern which, almost regardless of its shape, provoked a pattern of doctor behaviour which barely seemed to change.

Thus, concentrating upon the behaviours observed in Chapters 4, 5, 6 and 7 we tried to produce a simple and short check list. None of these attempts were successful because every effort to shorten or simplify the list reduced the sensitivity of the instrument to the range of behaviours commonly observed in a consultation.

* See pages 106 & 146.

What we were able to observe about a large range of consultations was the following:

1. There are behaviours which stem from the doctor's need to "know" (ie a clear understanding of symptoms).
2. There are those behaviours which stem from the doctor's need to "control" (ie to limit the patient to a defined area).
3. There are those behaviours which stem from the recognition of the patient's undeclared needs (ie dealing with apparent anxieties).
4. There are those behaviours which stem from a belief in the ability of the patient to make decisions and to be involved in his own treatment.

None of these four observations places an absolute value upon any particular behaviour. There are some behaviours in which the doctor's need to control is less manifest than in others. Equally, there are behaviours which are less capable of producing patient responses than others.

Two sets of tests have been developed from the details of behaviour, the first of which is presented overleaf:

This is our original doctor behaviour check list. It lists all of the behaviours we identified in the earlier chapters and is arranged in three areas:

Doctor-centred behaviour
Patient-centred behaviour
Negative behaviour.

These three lists were the result of many attempts to order the various lists so that a more coherent system of analysis could be developed. Taking the four observations made above it was possible to group behaviours around 1 and 2 which are essentially doctor-centred (in that they relate to the needs of the doctor), and then to group some behaviours around 3 and 4 which are patient-centred (ie that they relate to the doctor's perception of the patient's need to express his needs).

The negative behaviours are a group on their own and are not listed as being "doctor-" or "patient-centred". They should, on the whole, be placed in "doctor centered" behaviours because they are used to defend the doctor against his patient. Individual units of this type of behaviour occur in the majority of consultations. As we shall show, in the analysis of a consultation, it is normal to record occasional uses of negative behaviour. What is not normal is to find that the majority of behaviour is found in that area.

In the development of our analysis some of the behaviours have been placed in one of the three areas when there could be good arguments for placing them elsewhere. During three experiments to define this first check list "reassurance" changed its position three times. It is still possible to argue that reassurance has more to do with the needs of the doctor to contain emotion in his patient than it has to do with the patient's own needs. What we observe about reassurance is that much of it seems to have the desired effect, which should mean that the effect of the behaviour is patient-centred.

"Miscellaneous professional noises" present a problem. It is often difficult to distinguish between some grunts which are no more than professional grunts and other grunts which are an encouragement to the patient to keep talking. It has to be remembered that physical examinations can take place at the same time as a verbal examination. The only way in which a decision can be made by an external observer is to examine the context and effect of the various noises.

Doctors Name _____   Ref No ____   Patient Data M [ ] F [ ]   SC [1 | 2 | 3 | 4 | 5]

Doctor Centered Behaviour

Offering self					
Relating to some previous experience					
Directing					
Direct question					
Closed question					
Self answering question (Rhetorical)					
Placing events in time or sequence or place					
Correlational question					
Clarifying					
Doubting					
Chastising					
Justifying other agencies					
Criticising other agencies					
Challenging					
Summarising to close off					
Repeating what patient said for affirmation					
Giving information or opinion					
Advising					
Terminating (direct)					
Suggesting					
Apologising					
Misc Prof noises					
Suggesting or accepting collaboration					

Patient Centered Behaviour

Giving or seeking recognition					
Offering observation					
Broad question or opening					
Concealed question					
Encouraging					
Reflecting					
Exploring					
Answering patient question					
Accepting patient ideas					
Using patient ideas					
Offering of feeling					
Accepting feeling					
Using silence					
Summarising to open up					
Seeking patient ideas					
Reassuring					
Terminating (indirect)					
Indicating understanding					
Pre-directional probing					

Negative Behaviour

Rejecting patient offers					
Reinforcing self position (Justifying self)					
Denying patient					
Refusing patient ideas					
Evading patient questions					
Refusing to respond to feeling					
Not listening					
Confused noise					

Phase. [I | II. | III | IV | V. | VI]

146

If the effect is to keep a patient talking then they can be listed as "encouraging"; if the effect and context is such that the doctor makes no reaction to anything said by the patient then they may be listed as "miscellaneous professional noises"; in this case perhaps a charitable term.

"Clarifying" is sometimes difficult to distinguish from "reflecting". It may also, on occasion, be difficult to distinguish from "exploring". The whole point about "reflecting" and "exploring" is the way in which the patient is dictating the pace of the consultation and is merely being kept on course by the doctor. A "clarification" will refer to something said or done in the past (usually the immediate past of the proceeding consultation) and will only rarely form part of any future interaction between doctor and patient.

We have noted that occasionally some of our doctor guinea-pigs reacted badly to some of the placings and insisted that certain behaviours be placed in another category. We must accept that the ones referred to above are, in particular, open to debate. Anyone who feels strongly on any of these behaviours is free to move individual units around on the basis of reasoned argument. Behaviours such as a "direct question" cannot be "patient-centred" behaviour, any more than "reflecting" can be "doctor-centred" behaviour.

Progressing to the use which may be made of this instrument, here is a consultation involving a doctor and a patient who had arrived very late one evening to see this doctor's partner. The partner was away playing golf and this doctor was on his way out to a dinner party when his receptionist told him there was a patient in the waiting-room.

He was handed the case notes on which his partner had written "beware— garrulous old B——". We have indicated the doctor's behaviours in the bracketed comments.

D. "Come in. Do sit down." (Directing.) "Sorry to keep you waiting." (Apologising.) "Mr W——?"
P. "Yeah."
D. "Do sit down." (Directing.) "Ah, yes?" (Broad opening.)
P. "I hit my leg at work and went up to the infirmary last Wednesday and they dressed it and gave me needles and I think one at the infirmary ever since. I came up Thursday for a doctor's note and I got one, I think it was Dr R——."
D. "Yes." (Indicating understanding.)
P. "And it expires today."
D. "So you need another one." (Suggesting.)
P. "Yes."
D. "How bad is your leg now?" (Direct question.) "Is it properly dressed?" (Closed question.)
P. "I got another dressing to put on myself you see. I have to go again on Monday."
D. "Yes." (Indicating understanding.)
P. "The swelling's gone down, yesterday."
D. "Yes." (Encouraging.)
P. "But there's still a soreness, round my bum and that."
D. "Yes." (Encouraging.)
P. "It's in a bad spot."
D. "And you have to go back on Monday." (Repeating for affirmation.)

147

Doctors Name [ ] **Ref No** [ ] **Patient Data** [M | F] **SC** [1 | 2 | 3 | 4 | 5] **Age** 57

Doctor Centered Behaviour

Behaviour	Score
Offering self	
Relating to some previous experience	III
Directing	I
Direct question	I
Closed question	
Self answering question (Rhetorical)	
Placing events in time or sequence or place	
Correlational question	
Clarifying	
Doubting	
Chastising	
Justifying other agencies	
Criticising other agencies	
Challenging	
Summarising to close off	
Repeating what patient said for affirmation	I
Giving information or opinion	
Advising	
Terminating (direct)	I
Suggesting	I
Apologising	I
Misc Prof noises	I
Suggesting or accepting collaboration	

Patient Centered Behaviour

Behaviour	Score
Giving or seeking recognition	
Offering observation	
Broad question or opening	I
Concealed question	
Encouraging	II
Reflecting	
Exploring	
Answering patient question	
Accepting patient ideas	
Using patient ideas	
Offering of feeling	
Accepting feeling	
Using silence	
Summarising to open up	
Seeking patient ideas	
Reassuring	
Terminating (indirect)	
Indicating understanding	III
Pre-directional probing	

Negative Behaviour

Behaviour	Score
Rejecting patient offers	
Reinforcing self position (Justifying self)	
Denying patient	
Refusing patient ideas	
Evading patient questions	
Refusing to respond to feeling	
Not listening	
Confused noise	

Phase: [I | II | III | IV | V | VI]

148

This same doctor, scored over 18 consultations, produced an overall score which follows:

COMPOSITE SCORE

Doctors Name: L.J Ref No: ____ SC ____ Patient Data: M ____ F ____ 1 2 3 4 5 Age ____

Doctor Centered Behaviour

Behaviour	Tally	Score
Offering self		
Relating to some previous experience	卌 卌 卌 卌 卌 I	36
Directing	卌 卌 卌 卌 卌	25
Direct question	卌 卌 卌 卌 II	22
Closed question		
Self answering question (Rhetorical)		
Placing events in time or sequence or place	卌 卌 卌 卌	20
Correlational question	卌 卌 卌 卌 卌	25
Clarifying	卌 卌 卌	15
Doubting	卌	5
Chastising		
Justifying other agencies	III	3
Criticising other agencies		
Challenging	I	1
Summarising to close off		
Repeating what patient said for affirmation	卌 卌 卌 II	17
Giving information or opinion	卌 卌 卌 卌 IIII	24
Advising	卌 卌	10
Terminating (direct)	卌 卌 卌	15
Suggesting	卌 卌 卌 IIII	19
Apologising	卌 I	6
Misc Prof noises	卌 卌 卌 卌 卌 II	27
Suggesting or accepting collaboration		

Patient Centered Behaviour

Behaviour	Tally	Score
Giving or seeking recognition	III	4
Offering observation	卌	5
Broad question or opening	卌 卌 卌 卌	20
Concealed question	II	2
Encouraging	卌 卌 卌 卌 卌 I	26
Reflecting	II	2
Exploring		
Answering patient question	卌	5
Accepting patient ideas	I	1
Using patient ideas	I	1
Offering of feeling	II	2
Accepting feeling		
Using silence	II	2
Summarising to open up	II	2
Seeking patient ideas	I	1
Reassuring	卌 卌 卌 卌	20
Terminating (indirect)	卌	5
Indicating understanding	卌 卌 卌 卌 卌 卌 III	35
Pre-directional probing	卌	5

Negative Behaviour

Behaviour	Tally	Score
Rejecting patient offers		
Reinforcing self position (Justifying self)		
Denying patient		
Refusing patient ideas	卌 II	7
Evading patient questions	I	1
Refusing to respond to feeling	I	1
Not listening	III	3
Confused noise	卌 卌 卌	15

Phase: I | II | III | IV | V | VI

149

P. "Monday. On Monday."

D. "Yes." (Miscellaneous professional noises.)

P. "And, of course, I have to have another needle in five weeks time, you know."

D. "Oh, yes." (Indicating understanding.)

P. "Can I . . . ?"

D. "Here you are." (Terminating.) "Make an appointment for next Tuesday, will you?" (Directing.)*

This analysis has been used to examine nearly 1,000 of the consultations we have collected. As part of this analysis we were able to compare sets of consultations provided by 20 doctors, in which one set of consultations was provided for a complete morning surgery and a follow-up set of consultations was provided for a complete morning surgery some weeks later. Very little difference could be observed between the two sets. A rank order correlation of doctor-centred behaviours revealed that the range of positive correlation between the two sets ran from 0·73 to 0·81. The inference is, therefore, that doctors use the same behaviours in nearly the same order of preference. Similar results were obtained from the same test being applied to patient-centred behaviour (0·69 to 0·82).

This data goes a long way to support the hypotheses we have already dealt with in earlier chapters that doctors are remarkably consistent in the ways in which they consult with patients.

With a composite score sheet covering 20 or more consultations it is possible to consider this as the basis of a training programme. We have used this sort of analysis on many occasions and the last part of this chapter is a report on a pilot experiment we conducted in 1973–74 to ascertain the viability of our approach. Before we progress to that report let us examine a complete teaching situation we have undertaken with the doctor who figures in the composite score sheet on page 149.

The extract from a consultation we are going to examine was selected by the doctor himself as being the consultation which caused him most concern.

In this extract the patient had already offered the symptoms of severe headaches and a recurrent rash. He also had a history of various mild nervous disorders culminating two years previously in a quite severe ulceration of the stomach. The doctor knew that the patient was under considerable stress but had been unable to identify the cause. Over the past three years the doctor tried seven different prescriptions, none of which alleviated the condition but, equally, no real deterioration was evident in the patient. That a complete physical examination revealed no new information came as no surprise to the doctor. Again, our comments are in brackets.

D. "Now then, that all seems to be okay." (Reassurance.) "Get your shirt on and sit down." (Best described as a transitional direction.) "Now, tell me, are you under a lot of pressure at work?" (This looks like a direct question, but we consider it to be a concealed suggestion.)

---

*What follows has been listed as "terminating". It is fair to say that the doctor behaves as though the patient has not started to speak. An additional interpretation might well be "Not listening".

P. "No. I'm well on top of that now. I've given up altogether those late nights. I still take a little work home at nights, but I don't spend more than an hour at it. I have a little sleep between six and seven and I'm fresh as a daisy."

D. "Yes, but at work are you still under the same amount of pressure as you were last year? You know, when we had you in hospital you were pretty bad. Let's face it, your work was really on top of you then." (The doctor is still in the process of suggesting to the patient the cause of his problems.)

P. "No. You see, when I went back they gave me a new assistant. He's a nice lad. He has a day a week off to go to college and this seems to suit him. He's taken a load off me, you know. He earns his bread, does that lad. I expect he'll stay with us for the three years."

D. "What sort of schedule do you work to now? I mean, are you getting lunch, for example?" (A common surgery error on which we have previously commented. The doctor asks a fairly "broad question" but then closes off most of the patient's potential answers with a "closed question".)

P. "Oh, yes. Lunch for me is now one till two. I even get about ten minutes with my eyes closed."

D. "Ah-ha, so you are tired, then." (Finally classified as a "challenge".)

P. "No. If it's fine I get out and stroll around the grass for ten minutes. But it seems to rain more here than anywhere else. So I put my feet up."

D. "Well, how are things at home, then? How are your relationships with your wife? Have these suffered at all in the last few years?" (Although these three questions would be classified as "broad question" followed by two "direct questions" the effect again is suggestive.)

P. "Do you know, I think I have a very happy home. I don't have much to compare it with, but I think as homes go mine is pretty good."

D. "Well, do you have arguments with your wife? These can be very disturbing, you know." (Suggestion.)

P. "Argue with Mary? You asked me that before. I told her, you know, and we had a good laugh over that. I don't think we've had a cross word in ten years."

D. "How about the children?" (Broad question.)

P. "The oldest girl is doing an extra year at college, you know. She wants to be a teacher. I keep telling her there's no money in that, but these youngsters know their own minds, don't they?"

D. "What is John doing now?" (Direct question.)

P. "We finally got him settled in the tech you know. He seems to prefer that to the grammar school."

D. "So the family seems to be all well." (Summarising to close off.)

This consultation was discussed by a small group of four doctors who were set the task of enabling the doctor concerned to analyse the reason for his concern. Gradually he began to realise that what he had been trying to do was to think of all the possible causes of stress he had encountered. He was then offering these to the patient in an attempt to short-cut the consultation, hoping that what he considered to be a cause of stress would conveniently fit the patient. All of his short cuts, however, turned out to be dead ends. Referring to his composite score sheet he realised that he used "suggesting" very frequently.

151

In this consultation he decided that "suggesting" had not really helped him or the patient because the effect had been to cause the patient to refute the doctor's suggestions. He thus set himself the learning goal of reducing the amount of "suggesting" he used and increasing the amount of "exploring".

The training task was thus to devise a situation in which these goals might be pursued. Initially, the doctor was given examples of "exploring" and was invited to discuss with the trainers (B. E. L. Long and C. M. Harris) any questions he might have about the examples we provided. Following this we examined, in detail, his actual consultation to identify points at which he might have used some form of "exploration". Two possible areas emerged from this discussion—firstly, the patient's feelings about his work and, secondly, his feelings about his son.

In both cases we then referred back to the points in the transcript where possible alternative courses of action seemed possible. The first of these was the point where the patient replied:
P. "No. If it's fine I get out and stroll around the grass. . . ."

At this point in the transcript the doctor, as can be seen, moves away from the issue of work to consider the family. In the training situation the doctor was asked to hold the work issue in mind and try to find a form of words which might cause the patient to talk a little more about work. He produced the following "exploration":

"What do you think about when you are strolling around the grass?"

To this the trainer has to produce a response which will give the trainee the courage and motivation to proceed a little further. What we said was, naturally, a trainer's fantasy of what the patient might say and had no basis in any particular knowledge we had of the case:
Trainer: "Oh, about work. The morning and what has happened."
Trainee: "What happens in mornings which comes to mind?"
Trainer: "Oh, maybe it has been very boring, you know."

On the question of the son we used the following statement by the patient:
"He seems to prefer that to the grammar school."
Trainee: "Was he not happy at grammar school?"
Trainer: "Well, he used to skip school, you know."
Trainee: "Tell me more about that."

In this particular case we are fortunate enough to have some feedback from the doctor. He wrote a letter to one of us in which he enthused over his new-found skill. He had not found a solution, but he had found a potential cause of his patient's problems. It transpired that the guess about work was, in part, accurate. The patient had for a long time been considering giving up his job because he had, for many years, wished to become a social worker. The more he thought about becoming a social worker the less he liked his job. His job, however, was highly paid and he realised that to achieve his ambition he would have to take a substantial drop in income and he could not afford it. Rather to our chagrin the doctor did add that he had suggested that his patient look at the personnel management aspect of his work. The doctor was still being directive.

This approach to the learning of new behaviours has been the subject of a series of experiments conducted in the UK and in Australasia. In order to use the approach it might help the potential trainer to read about a very valuable insight gained in Australia whilst actually running such a programme.

One particular doctor decided to examine a consultation in which, he believed, his performance was at its worst. Based upon his own analysis of this particular consultation, he then set about examining each of his behaviours and postulated a set of alternative (and by his own definition and for his own purposes "more desirable") behaviours.

What he discovered was that his selection of new behaviours did not produce a behaviour which was blank in the composite score. Instead, what he found was that he was selecting behaviours which had collected two or three scores in his total set of analysed consultations. On reflection, a simple explanation is possible. Doctors, when selecting what they like to think of as "new" behaviours, will tend to select behaviours which they already have, although the incidence of usage of these behaviours is low. The doctor is reducing his risk factor in two ways. Firstly, he is reducing the learning effort required to learn a "new" behaviour and secondly, and perhaps more importantly, the doctor is reducing the risk he will have to take with his patients because the outcome of this known behaviour is already partly familiar—and thus more susceptible to control.

If one is in a trainer role the urge to step in at this point to impose some sort of reappraisal of the trainee's selection is enormous. Such urges, on the whole, should be resisted. In our scheme the purpose of a trainer is not to tell a trainee what he needs to learn but to help him learn those things which he decides to learn. This is, of course, a particular philosophic position we have taken vis-à-vis teachers and learners—trainers and trainees—and we have dealt with this point at length in "Learning to Care".[10]

The position we take is not exclusively based upon philosophic precept but equally upon observations which one can make about good teaching.

The objective of this particular form of teaching is to ensure that the learner utilises his learning in a real situation. Whilst it might well be gratifying for the teacher to hear the learner produce "desirable" responses in the learning situation, this is only half of the battle. The fact that the learner can, in controlled conditions, produce apt responses must not be taken to mean he will produce the same responses in real life situations.

Consequently, if a learner decides that he will select a particular level of learning which may, in the teacher's mind, be little more than minimal, the teacher must accept that, for the time being, this is what he himself should be concerned with. To attempt to impose more on the learner than he is ready or willing to accept is to reduce the value of the learning situation.

There are certain distinct advantages in accepting the level of learning prescribed by the learner. The most obvious one is the probability of success. Success has a remarkable effect on motivation. Learners who achieve a particular level of learning will be more willing, and often capable, to learn at a new higher level.

For those interested in training technique what we have done is to combine a feature of a relatively new teaching technique (micro-teaching) and a relatively old technique (role-playing). The basis of micro-teaching is an analysis of patterns of behaviour a teacher might use in a classroom. In our case we have compiled a list of behaviours a doctor might use in his consulting-room. To this we have added the idea of role-playing a variety of different situations in which the learner is required to experiment with those forms of behaviour he wishes to acquire. The role-play, however, is not a complete acting out of a full consultation, but is based upon small excerpts from consultations which the learner has actually produced himself.

The teaching mechanism then is simple. It requires no great expertise for an experienced GP to place himself in the position of a patient, particularly when the lead lines of the script are already provided.

In an attempt to evaluate the potential of this approach we ran a pilot experiment in which we decided to measure the learning gain of a group of teachers of general practice provided with the method by means of a course. A report on part of this pilot experiment has already been published in *Der Praktische Arzt*.

A summary of the research paper is appended.

The research design

Note: The word "trainer" is used below to mean the two people who ran the course.

1. Tape recordings of at least one complete surgery were made by each participant one month prior to attending the residential course.
2. These tapes were analysed utilising the behaviour check list.
3. On entry to the programme each participant was given an analysis of his behaviour and style (see composite check list) and was invited to compare the trainer's perception of his tapes with his own perception of them.
4. The course members were split into groups and each group reviewed all its members' tapes and analyses.
5. Differences of opinion related to the analyses were discussed between the trainers and the individual course members and also between the course members and the individuals.
6. Each course member was given a period of time to consider his style and behaviour and to decide which new behaviours he wished to adopt.
7. Each course member declared his learning goals to the trainers and to his own group. The trainers and each group then devised a total series of *inter-active* experiments which would allow each individual course member to practice specific behaviours.
8. One week after leaving the programme each member returned a new tape of a full surgery for analysis by the trainers.
9. Six months after the course each member returned a new tape of another full surgery for analysis.
10. Four doctors volunteered to act as a control group and returned tapes before the programme and approximately at the same time as each set of post-course tapes were returned.

Experimental limitations

1. Only seven of the original 15 course members provided complete required data.

   Only 11 of the 15 provided two-thirds of the required data.

   This paper is thus only an indication of a direction rather than a complete piece of research analysis.

Summary of findings
1. All but one of the course members displayed strong patterns of "doctor-centred" behaviour and presented their personal learning goal as "the learning of more patient-centred behaviour".
2. All of the first recall tapes (one week post-course) demonstrated a 15 to 20 per cent increase in "patient-centred" behaviour and the lengthening of consultation times by up to 20 per cent.
3. In most cases, however, the same quantity of "doctor-centred" behaviour was observed and the "patient-centred" behaviour had been grafted on— hence the increase in time.
4. Of the final seven tapes, four demonstrated that the "patient-centred" behaviour was becoming more naturally incorporated into the consultation. But the increment in "patient-centred" behaviour had dropped from 20 to 8 per cent.
5. In terms of consulting styles (see Chapter 9 ff) all four sets of "improved tapes" showed a continued movement of style along the patient-centred axis. The other three showed an initial movement of style in the first post-course tape, but the final tape demonstrated a reversion to the sender's previous style.

Detail
First tapes (after discussion with students)
A total in excess of 2,000 units of doctor behaviour were examined in this experiment. These were derived from seven doctors. In the control group (four doctors) a total of 1,200 units of behaviour was examined. In the control group no significant differences were discovered in any of the recorded consultations except with one doctor on the first retest. This doctor, who has a patient participative style when achieving a diagnosis, with a strong prescriptive style, suddenly changed his pattern and became very authoritarian and "doctor-centred". He subsequently explained that he was aware of this change and ascribed it to the pressure of patients in the waiting-room. He also claims to be unhappy when he felt he was forced to take this approach and considered that he was a less effective doctor when doing so.

Table 1 *Analysis of total group behaviours in the experiment* (as scored by the trainers)

Doctor-centred	77%
Patient-centred	21%
Negative	5%
Collaborative	1·5%

NB. Approximately 5 per cent of tapes lost due to recording failures and poor tape quality.

The next table is the analysis of the same data performed by the course members themselves. In brackets the original scores offered by the researcher trainers:

Doctor-centred	73·5	(77)
Patient-centred	23·5	(21)
Negative	2·0	(0·5)
Collaborative	1·0	(1·5)

155

The major area of disagreement was in the area of "negative" behaviour. The researchers had scored these as "non-listening noises" eg various grunts and "mmms". The doctor, however, felt that these were important encouragements to the patient.

(Dr C. M. Harris also scored several tapes and produced results which differed with the interpretations of the researcher by up to 5 per cent. It does seem that at least 5 per cent of all judgements will be open to question, and this may well constitute an error factor in this part of the research.)

One area which causes severe problems is that of "miscellaneous professional noises", the various grunts made by doctors when conducting a verbal examination. These are not as difficult to interpret as when the doctor is also examining the patient physically.

Some doctors claim that they make the noises to show the patient that they are doing something; others claim the noises are made to reassure patients; and others claim that each noise indicates the closure of some part of the physical examination. In this research all such noises were labelled "miscellaneous professional noises." (Doctor-centred.)

Table 2 *Quantification of "noise" made by doctor and patients in consultations prior to the experiment*

	Experimental group	Control group
Total doctor noise	29%	31%
Total patient noise	50%	52%
Total silence	13%	7%
Total confused noise	5%	9%
Loss due to poor tape	3%	1%

This table is an analysis of the actual noise (or absence of noise) made by the two parties in a consultation. For three or four person consultations in which more than one person was present, in addition to the doctor, both the patient and the accompanying person(s) have been scored as patient noise. It is worth noting that the bulk of the confused noise is to be found in consultations involving more than two persons.

Table 3 *First post-experiment test (one week)*

	Experiment	Control
Total doctor noise	22%	36%
Total patient noise	47%	53%
Total silence	29%	6%
Total confused noise	2%	5%
Loss	0%	2%

This is perhaps a startling result due to the large increase in the duration of silence. This can be, in the main, ascribed to two factors. Firstly, "silence" as a therapeutic tool was emphasised on the course and many of the course members expressed an interest in its value. Secondly, patients used to behaving in a particular way were undoubtedly confused by the doctor's change in style. One patient actually asked a doctor why he was remaining quiet for so long. The consultation proceeded as follows:

D. "I have just been on a course where we were studying the ways in which silence helps a patient and the doctor."

156

P. "It makes you think, doesn't it?"

Quite what was being thought, sadly, was never made explicit.

Table 4   *Second-post experiment test (six months)*

	Experiment	Control
Total doctor noise	24%	34%
Total patient noise	54%	52%
Total silence	20%	8%
Total confused noise	1%	5%
Loss	1%	1%

The silence factor is clearly declining, but significantly the "confused noise" element has stayed at a low level. The silence factor is still, however, significantly greater than at the start and remains higher than in the control group. Unfortunately the value of the data from the control group is diluted in the second recall, because only two interviews were conducted with more than one person in the consulting-room and consequently the opportunities to create confused noise were not the same.

There is here some prima facie evidence to suggest that there is a casual relationship between a course which concentrates upon factors such as "listening" and "using silence" and the manifestation of these phenomena in subsequent consultations.

Behaviour learning

The seven doctors who have been followed through the complete experiment postulated that they would like to learn the use of the following behaviours:

Encouraging
Using patient ideas
Reflecting
Broad question
Summarising to open up
Seeking patient ideas.

(In the original group of 17 a further 12 behaviours were listed, but these tapes have not been analysed because of the incomplete nature of the returns.)

Table 5 *Incidence of "new" behaviours noted during three tests (seven doctors) compared with a control group of four doctors*

	E1 (pretest)	E2 (1 week)	E3 (6 months)	C1	C2	C3
Encouraging	45	70	61	21	17	23
Using patient ideas	12	26	17	7	12	11
Reflecting	7	19	12	3	0	1
Broad questions	30	37	43	12	11	13
Summary to open up	2	7	9	0	2	1
Seeking patient ideas	18	21	23	6	8	8
	114	180	165	49	50	57
(÷ 7)	$16\frac{3}{7}$	$25\frac{5}{7}$	$23\frac{5}{7}$	$12\frac{1}{4}$	$12\frac{1}{2}$	$14\frac{1}{4}$ (÷ 4)

We have already noted the increase in silence, and stated that the use of silence was listed as a learning objective. On this set of data we note that the

157

experimental group were already using the behaviours indicated more frequently than were their control counterparts. As might be expected the pattern of increase in the first post-test is markedly greater than one finds some weeks later. However, what has been retained is interesting. The most difficult behaviour in the list is undoubtedly "reflecting". It is difficult for two reasons. Firstly, judging when it may be useful and, secondly, because it can produce no response at all in the patient. Obviously, its use must have produced problems. Whilst it shows a great increase on the first retest it is markedly down on the second. "Using patient ideas" is also difficult if only because many of the ideas produced may well not accord with desirable medical objectives. This behaviour, too, seems to have been over-used in the first retest but has been placed into a more sober perspective by the second.

Although there is such a small control group, one interesting hypothesis emerges which might be worth testing in depth. Where there already exist behaviours there can be an increment in their quantity without any form of training, *vide* "using patient ideas" and "seeking patient ideas". Another interesting factor in the control group concerns one member who had, three years previously, attended a course on counselling where he had learned something of "reflecting". If we eliminate him from the control group that particular behaviour does not appear at all. This would suggest that there are a number of useful behaviours which may be learned on a course that otherwise would never be learned.

Taken with the previous data in Tables 2, 3 and 4 this evidence is certainly worth more investigation because all of these behaviours will predictably cause a silence—simply because they require a patient to think harder. The balance in the consultations is shifting more than marginally towards the patient, even though the most significant factor in the consultations is the quantity of silence and the reduction in confused noise.

Consultation time (in minutes)

Average times by doctor

Doctor	Experimental group			Control group		
	Pretest	1st recall	2nd recall	Pretest	1st recall	2nd recall
1	6·2	7·3 (+ 1·1)	7·0 (+ 0·8)	6·3	6·6	6·6
2	5·7	6·8 (+ 1·1)	6·2 (+ 0·5)	4·5	5·0	4·9
3	7·1	8·0 (+ 0·9)	7·9 (+ 0·8)	6·4	6·6	5·8
4	6·8	6·8 (0)	7·2 (+ 0·4)	5·5	5·8	5·9
5	4·7	4·3 (− 0·4)	4·8 (+ 0·1)			
6	5·1	8·5 (+ 3·4)	7·6 (+ 2·5)			
7	5·9	7·0 (+ 1·1)	7·8 (+ 1·9)			

There is some evidence here that consultation times have actually increased from a minimum of six seconds up to a maximum of two-and-a-half minutes. Much of the increase may be accounted for by the increase in the amount of silence and the decrease in the quantity of time the doctor uses, compared with the increase in the quantity of time the patient has been permitted to use.

What is apparent, however, is that using these new behaviours does increase the amount of time actually spent with individual patients. Unfortunately, we have no data to allow us to speculate on whether patients then come back for fewer consultations than previously. Over the whole group there is an average increase of one minute per patient, which could mean an addition of more than

20 to 30 minutes to a normal surgery. If we take the high point of the range, however, the possibility exists of an increment of almost 50 per cent to a surgery schedule time.

Conclusions

On the whole all the conclusions from this experiment must be tentative because the numbers are so small. As one would expect, the gains are not sustained in most cases, but the rate of "relapse" to the previous norm is not as high as might have been predicted. Clearly, the course did have a distinct effect in terms of providing something of what the course members wished to learn. No judgement may be made here of desirable clinical outcomes because the researcher is not qualified to make such judgements. The experiment itself was an experiment in teaching and learning and it is as such that it must be judged. The only judgement made is that of the participants in the experiment, who clearly themselves have shown that they valued some of that which they learned.

In order to examine the methodology a similar experiment was conducted on nurse students. In that experiment a group of behaviours was indicated as "desirable", but the learning process was the same. In a well controlled experiment an increment on "desirable" behaviours in excess of 100 per cent was achieved. We thus conclude that the methodology itself is basically valid as a means of developing behaviours.

CHAPTER 14

THE MEASUREMENTS OF CONSULTING STYLES: A "DO-IT-YOURSELF" KIT

In the previous chapter we were examining the overall pattern of behaviour units a doctor uses in a complete set of 20 consultations. The use of such information in training was discussed largely in terms of ways in which individual units of behaviour might be incorporated into the overall pattern of behaviours displayed by a doctor. It was also indicated that such an instrument could also be used to demonstrate that some behaviours were over-utilised and others were under-utilised.

This final chapter is designed to use a similar pattern of information generated by the same type of examination of consultations apart from the fact that we are now going to break the consultation into two parts. Firstly, we are going to examine those behaviours which occur before that point in a consultation at which the doctor appears to have made a decision about the condition of the patient. Subsequently, we are going to examine those behaviours which occur after that point.

In Chapters 10 and 11 we concluded that consultations appeared to fall into four basic styles of diagnosis and seven basic styles of prescription. We have, so far, made no attempt to quantify a style apart from indicating in Chapters 10 and 11 those behaviours which appear to be predominant in any particular style. Originally it was hoped that the information we needed on the question of style could be elicited simply by inspection. Utilising transcripts and the check list of behaviours we introduced in the last chapter it is possible to make a crude assessment.

During the preparation of the material used as the basis of Chapters 10 and 11 we examined 10 consecutive consultations by 15 different doctors. Each of these consultations was broken into two parts around that point at which it appeared that the doctor had made a decision and was preparing to move the consultation forward into prescription. All of the consultations were examined and scored according to the check list. Subsequent inspection produced the following data, which represents a set of judgements made by the researcher about each of the consultations. In the first column the scores may range from 1 to 4 (ie the four diagnostic styles) and the second column from 1 to 7 (ie prescriptive styles).

The results are as follows:

Dr A.	1,1,1,1,2,1,2,1,1,1.	2,3,2,3,3,2,2,2,2,2.
Dr B.	1,1,1,1,1,1,1,1,1,1.	1,1,1,1,1,2,2,4,1,1.
Dr C.	1,1,1,1,3,1,3,1,1,1.	2,2,2,2,1,3,3,6,1,1.
Dr D.	2,2,2,2,2,2,2,1,2,1.	3,3,3,3,3,3,4,2,1,3.
Dr E.	1,1,1,1,1,1,1,1,2,1.	1,1,1,1,1,1,1,1,1,2.
Dr F.	2,2,2,2,2,2,2,4,2,2.	4,4,3,4,3,4,3,3/2,3,3.
Dr G.	3,3,3,2,3,4,3,3,3,1.	1,1,1,1,1,1,1,1,1,1.
Dr H.	1,1,1,1,2,1,1,2,1,1.	1,2,2,1,2,2,2,2,1,2.
Dr J.	2,3,2,3,2,3,1,2,3,2.	5,5,5,5,5,5,4,5,4,1,5.
Dr K.	1,1,1,1,1,1,1,2,1,2.	1,1,1,1,1,1,2,1,2,2.
Dr L.	3,4,3,3,3,3,3,3,3,1.	4,5,6,6,6,4,6,4,5,5.
Dr M.	1,2,1,2,2,2,2,2,1,2.	2,3,2,3,2,3,3,3,3,3.
Dr N.	2,3,2,3,3,3,3,3,3,3.	2,2,2,2,2,2,3,2,3,2.
Dr O.	1,1,1,1,1,1,2,1,2,2.	1,1,1,2,1,2,1,1,1,1.
Dr P.	1,2,2,2,2,2,1,2,1,2.	2,2,2,2,2,2,2,2,3,2.

Prima facie this appears to be a simple statement of style and range of style, but in fact it suffers from a number of weaknesses.

In the first place the description of styles in Chapters 10 and 11 are descriptions of stereotypes and as such can only be treated as broad indicators rather than something specific. Take the example of Dr B—— above. He would appear on inspection to be rigidly confined to a diagnostic style which gives little indication of any real flexibility. In fact, some of the judgements were very fine and had he used one or two more "encouraging noises" and one or two less "closed questions" then at least three of the consultations would have fallen into Style 2. Exactly the same comment may be made about Dr E——.

160

The problem is, therefore, to develop a measure which will enable a trainer to give a trainee a precise picture of his style and a picture of his existing potential range of styles.

The technique we have used to do this is to invest each unit of behaviour with a value which corresponds to the number of the style with which it is most closely associated. Consequently, if we identify a particular unit of behaviour as "chastising", that behaviour is most commonly to be found in consultations which, during the diagnostic phase, we have labelled Style 1. Hence "chastising" carries a score value of 1. "Encouraging", on the other hand, is more commonly found in Style 3 or 4, thus it earns a score value of $3\frac{1}{2}$.

The two check lists we have devised are not the same as the one we examined in the last chapter. It will be observed that the two have different titles. The first check list is of those behaviours which are most commonly found in the diagnostic phases of a consultation, and the second is a list of those behaviours most commonly found in the prescribing phases. The first list has a score range of 1 to 4, corresponding with the four styles of diagnosis we have identified, whilst the second list has a score range of 1 to 7, corresponding with the seven styles we have identified for prescribing.

The list of negative behaviours constitute a problem in this system because they do not commonly occur in any style with any degree of frequency. With the exception of a few consultations involving patients who were trying to extract drugs from doctors, or patients trying to have bottles of proprietary substances added to a prescription (eg Dettol), we have not been able to discover any evidence of a consistent negative style. We have, however, identified a number of negative behaviours which do occur in a large number of consultations. They do not appear with a high degree of frequency and they are, on the whole, used as a controlling device to prevent patients talking about matters the doctor does not wish to discuss. In order to score these we have decided that they should carry a negative score and, consequently, we have used a score range of minus 1 to minus 2.

Each of these two lists contains, as we said above, those behaviours which occur most commonly in any of the styles we have identified. Each of the lists contains behaviours not to be found in the other. The decision to eliminate or include is based upon the probability of a behaviour occurring in either of the two parts of the consultation. This, of course, does not mean that a particular behaviour may not occur there under any circumstances. For our purposes, however, should such a "rogue" behaviour be seen to occur it is simply not scored.

Some of the score values carry a score such as $2\frac{1}{2}$ or $3\frac{1}{2}$. The half score indicates that the behaviour may well occur naturally in two of the styles we have identified. Equally, a score of 2 or 3 can indicate that a behaviour occurs not only in Style 2 or 3 but in the styles on either side, ie 1 and 3 or 2 and 4.

Scoring method;

In order to score these sheets, a consultation must initially be divided into its two sections, ie before decision about patient and after decision. Again, it is valuable to have a transcript of the consultation, especially if the doctor has had to revert from a later phase to an earlier phase (eg from Phase V to Phase II,

CHECK LIST OF BEHAVIOURS WITH SCORE VALUES USED IN THE DIAGNOSTIC PHASES OF A CONSULTATION

Doctor Centered Behaviour	Score Value	Incidence	I x SV
Offering Self	1		
Relating to some previous experience	1½		
Direct question	1½		
Closed question	½		
Self answering question (Rhetorical)	½		
Placing events in time or sequence or place	2		
Correlational question	1½		
Clarifying	3		
Doubting	1½		
Chastising	1		
Justifying other agencies	1		
Criticising other agencies	1		
Challenging	2½		
Summarising to close off	1		
Repeating what patient said for affirmation	2		
Suggesting	1½		
Apologising	1½		
Misc. Prof. noises	1½		
Directing	1½		
Giving information or opinion	2		

Patient Centered Behaviour	Score Value	Incidence	I x SV
Giving or seeking recognition	1½		
Offering observation	3		
Broad question	2½		
Concealed question	3		
Encouraging	3		
Reflecting	4		
Exploring	2½		
Answering patient question	2		
Accepting patient ideas	4		
Using Patient ideas	3		
Offering of feeling	2½		
Accepting feeling	4		
Using silence	4		
Summarising to open up	3		
Seeking patient ideas	4		
Reassuring	1		
Indicating understanding	2½		

Negative Behaviour	Score Value	Indicence	I x SV
Rejecting patient offers	−1		
Reinforcing self position (justifying self)	−1		
Denying patient	−1		
Refusing patient ideas	−1		
Evading patient questions	−1		
Refusing to respond to feeling	−1		
Not listening	−2		
Confused noise	−1		

Doctor Centered Behaviour	Score Value	Incidence	I x SV
Relating to some previous experience	1½		
Directing	1½		
Clarifying	5½		
Doubting	3		
Chastising	2		
Justifying other agencies	1		
Criticising other agencies	1		
Challenging	4		
Summarising to close off	2		
Repeating what patient said for affirmation	3		
Giving information or opinion	3		
Advising	3½		
Terminating (direct)	1		
Suggesting	3		
Misc. Prof. noises	1		
Suggesting or accepting collaboration	4½		

Patient Centered Behaviour	Score Value	Incidence	I x SV
Offering observation	3½		
Broad question	3½		
Encouraging	5½		
Reflecting	6½		
Exploring	5½		
Answering patient question	4		
Accepting patient ideas	6		
Using patient ideas	4½		
Offering of feeling	4½		
Accepting feeling	5		
Using silence	7		
Summarising to open up	5½		
Seeking patient ideas	4½		
Reassuring	3		
Terminating (indirect)	4		
Indicating understanding	3		
Pre-directional probing	4½		

Negative Behaviour	Score Value	Incidence	I x SV
Rejecting patient offers	1		
Reinforcing self position (justifying self)	−1		
Denying Patient	−1		
Refusing Patient ideas	−1		
Evading patient questions	−1		
Refusing to respond to feeling	−1		
Not listening	−2		
Confused noise	−1		

163

see Chapter 3). A very common form of reverting is found when the doctor during Phase V asks a question such as:

"How old are you now?"

It may well be argued that such a question is wholly appropriate to Phase V behaviour and that it is being used to lead the patient towards a conclusion the doctor already has in mind—for example, confronting manual labourers that they cannot continue indefinitely with manual labour. It may, however, be equally argued that the information should already have been elicited in Phase II if it is not already written on the case notes in front of the doctor. A more appropriate Phase V behaviour would surely be:

"You know, you are now 55 are you not?"

which can then be classified as a "challenge" which seeks to confront the patient directly with the issue the doctor has in mind.

Let us examine two transcripts to see how they may be scored.

Example 1

D. "Come in Mr J——. How are things coming along?" (Giving recognition. Broad opening.)

P. "Oh, not too bad, doctor. I still have a little pain but things seem to be a lot easier."

D. "Good. How is the knee holding up?" (Direct question.)

P. "Fine. I have a little swelling around the ankle now."

D. "Let's have a look. Take your shoes and socks off and roll up the trouser leg." (Directing.)

P. "There, see?"

D. "Mmm. Mmm. Yes. I see. Mmm. Mmm." (Miscellaneous professional noise). "Move it around." (Directing.) "Good. Mmm. Mmm." (Miscellaneous professional noise.) "Fine, good. Right, roll it down and put your socks on. Right." (Directing and closing off.)

Fifteen second gap whilst patient dresses.

D. "Okay. When did this swelling come up?" (Placing events.)

P. "On Thursday."

D. "On Thursday." (Repeating what the patient said for affirmation.)

P. "Yes."

D. "Well, I don't think it is very serious. It's just a little strain due to you placing a lot of weight on that joint because of the way you are walking. When the knee eases up it will probably go away." (Giving information.)

P. "It's nothing serious then, is it?"

D. "No, not at all." (Answering patient question.) "Keep that bandage on the knee for a week or two more and if the ankle does not improve then come back in a fortnight. Okay?" (Directing. Summarising to close off.)

P. "Right you are then."

D. "Cheerio." (Terminating.)

This consultation divides easily after the reply to the question which was concerned to determine when the swelling had occurred. The doctor clearly moves into Phase IV (sharing information) and then quickly into Phase V and Phase VI.

This consulation would be scored on the two sheets as follows:

164

**CHECK LIST OF BEHAVIOURS WITH SCORE VALUES USED IN THE
DIAGNOSTIC PHASES OF A CONSULTATION**

Doctor Centered Behaviour	Score Value	Incidence	I x SV
Offering Self			
Relating to some previous experience			
Direct question	1½	1	1½
Closed question			
Self answering question (Rhetorical)			
Placing events in time or sequence or place	2	1	2
Correlational question			
Clarifying			
Doubting			
Chastising			
Justifying other agencies			
Criticising other agencies			
Challenging			
Summarising to close off	1	1	1
Repeating what patient said for affirmation	2	1	2
Suggesting			
Apologising			
Misc. Prof. noises	1½	11	3
Directing	1½	·111	4½
Giving information or opinion			

Patient Centered Behaviour	Score Value	Incidence	I x SV
Giving or seeking recognition	1½	1	1½
Offering observation			
Broad question	2½	1	2½
Concealed question			
Encouraging			
Reflecting			
Exploring			
Answering patient question			
Accepting patient ideas			
Using Patient ideas			
Offering of feeling			
Accepting feeling			
Using silence			
Summarising to open up			
Seeking patient ideas			
Reassuring			
Indicating understanding			

Negative Behaviour	Score Value	Incidence	I x SV
Rejecting patient offers			
Reinforcing self position (justifying self)			
Denying patient			
Refusing patient ideas			
Evading patient questions			
Refusing to respond to feeling			
Not listening			
Confused noise			

165

Doctor Centered Behaviour	Score Value	Incidence	I x SV
Relating to some previous experience			
Directing	1 ½	1	1 ½
Clarifying			
Doubting			
Chastising			
Justifying other agencies			
Criticising other agencies			
Challenging			
Summarising to close off	2	1	2
Repeating what patient said for affirmation			
Giving information or opinion	3	1	3
Advising			
Terminating (direct)	1	1	1
Suggesting			
Misc. Prof. noises			
Suggesting or accepting collaboration			

Patient Centered Behaviour	Score Value	Incidence	I x SV
Offering observation			
Broad question			
Encouraging			
Reflecting			
Exploring			
Answering patient question	4	1	4
Accepting patient ideas			
Using patient ideas			
Offering of feeling			
Accepting feeling			
Using silence			
Summarising to open up			
Seeking patient ideas			
Reassuring			
Terminating (indirect)			
Indicating understanding			
Pre-directional probing			

Negative Behaviour	Score Value	Incidence	I x SV
Rejecting patient offers			
Reinforcing self position (justifying self)			
Denying Patient			
Refusing Patient ideas			
Evading patient questions			
Refusing to respond to feeling			
Not listening			
Confused noise			

In the diagnostic phases the doctor used 11 units of behaviour. His total I. x S.V. score is 18. His diagnostic style may then be expressed as:

$$\frac{18}{11} = 1\cdot6$$

From this consultation we would therefore conclude that his style lay in between the stereotypes 1 and 2.

On the prescriptive sheet the doctor used five units of behaviour and his total I. x S.V. score is $11\frac{1}{2}$. This demonstrates a style which, at $2\cdot3$, lies in between prescribing styles 2 and 3.

This same doctor, over 10 consultations, produced the following scores:
Diagnostic:
  $1\cdot5$, $2\cdot0$, $1\cdot9$, $2\cdot1$, $2\cdot2$, $2\cdot3$, $2\cdot4$, $1\cdot6$, $2\cdot1$, $2\cdot2$.
Prescriptive:
  $3\cdot1$, $3\cdot2$, $2\cdot8$, $4\cdot2$, $4\cdot1$, $2\cdot6$, $3\cdot9$, $2\cdot3$, $3\cdot1$, $4\cdot3$.

Taking the total number of his behaviours and the total of his I. x S.V. score we find that he has a mean style of:
  $2\cdot15$ Diagnostic: with a range of $1\cdot5$–$2\cdot4$.
  $2\cdot7$ Prescriptive: with a range of $2\cdot3$–$4\cdot3$.

Example 2

D. "Hello, Mr W——. What can I do for you today?" (Giving recognition. Broad opening.)
P. "Well, I'm not too good you know."
D. "Tell me, then." (Finally classified as seeking patient ideas.)
P. "Well, I've got this pain in my ear. A sore throat and I keep losing my voice."
D. "Do you think you have a cold?" (Seeking patient ideas.)
P. "Oh. Oh, yes, I do."
D. "Mmm. Mmm. Go on." (Encouraging.)
P. "Well, I was up on the roof all yesterday, you know."
D. "On the roof? What were you doing there?" (Direct question.)
P. "Well, I was putting a new tile on. It was terribly cold."
D. "Go on." (Encouraging.)
P. "Well, last night I got this throat and then I started to have a bit of a sweat and then my voice went."
D. "Do you have a temperature? Have you taken it?" (Direct and closed question.)
P. "Aye. It's one hundred."
D. "Right, let's have a little look. Open wide." (Directing.) "Mmm." (Miscellaneous professional noise.) "Let's look at this ear. Turn a little, will you?" (Directing.) "Mmm. Mmm. Uh, hu. That's good." (Miscellaneous professional noise.) "Right you are, Mr. W——." (Closing off.)
P. "Thank you, doctor."
D. "Right, now. You are off home to bed for three days. On the way take this to the chemist. Take it three times a day after meals." (Directing.) "Nothing to worry about. It'll clear up quickly enough." (Reassuring.) "All right then? Cheerio." (Terminating.)

This consultation is scored on the following pages.

CHECK LIST OF BEHAVIOURS WITH SCORE VALUES USED IN THE DIAGNOSTIC PHASES OF A CONSULTATION

Doctor Centered Behaviour	Score Value	Incidence	I x SV
Offering Self			
Relating to some previous experience			
Direct question	1½	1 1	3
Closed question	½	1	½
Self answering question (Rhetorical)			
Placing events in time or sequence or place			
Correlational question			
Clarifying			
Doubting			
Chastising			
Justifying other agencies			
Criticising other agencies			
Challenging			
Summarising to close off	1	1	1
Repeating what patient said for affirmation			
Suggesting			
Apologising			
Misc. Prof. noises	1½	1 1	3
Directing	1½	1 1	3
Giving information or opinion			

Patient Centered Behaviour	Score Value	Incidence	I x SV
Giving or seeking recognition	1½	1	1½
Offering observation			
Broad question	2½	1	2½
Concealed question			
Encouraging	3	1 1	6
Reflecting			
Exploring			
Answering patient question			
Accepting patient ideas			
Using Patient ideas			
Offering of feeling			
Accepting feeling			
Using silence			
Summarising to open up			
Seeking patient ideas	4	1 1	8
Reassuring			
Indicating understanding			

Negative Behaviour	Score Value	Incidence	I x SV
Rejecting patient offers			
Reinforcing self position (justifying self)			
Denying patient			
Refusing patient ideas			
Evading patient questions			
Refusing to respond to feeling			
Not listening			
Confused noise			

Doctor Centered Behaviour	Score Value	Incidence	I x SV
Relating to some previous experience			
Directing	1½	1	1½
Clarifying			
Doubting			
Chastising			
Justifying other agencies			
Criticising other agencies			
Challenging			
Summarising to close off			
Repeating what patient said for affirmation			
Giving information or opinion			
Advising			
Terminating (direct)	1	1	1
Suggesting			
Misc. Prof. noises			
Suggesting or accepting collaboration			

Patient Centered Behaviour	Score Value	Incidence	I x SV
Offering observation			
Broad question			
Encouraging			
Reflecting			
Exploring			
Answering patient question			
Accepting patient ideas			
Using patient ideas			
Offering of feeling			
Accepting feeling			
Using silence			
Summarising to open up			
Seeking patient ideas			
Reassuring	3	1	3
Terminating (indirect)			
Indicating understanding			
Pre-directional probing			

Negative Behaviour	Score Value	Incidence	I x SV
Rejecting patient offers			
Reinforcing self position (justifying self)			
Denying Patient			
Refusing Patient ideas			
Evading patient questions			
Refusing to respond to feeling			
Not listening			
Confused noise			

From this we see that his diagnostic style is fractionally greater than 2 and his prescribing style is fractionally greater than 1·8. Over 10 consultations this doctor produces the following data:

Diagnostic:

2·9, 2·8, 3·1, 2·7, 2·6, 3·1, 2·3, 1·9, 2·8, 2·6.

Prescribing:

1·8, 1·9, 2·2, 3·3, 2·9, 2·8, 3·1, 4·0, 3·3, 2·1.

His means are:

Diagnostic: 2·95   range 1·9–3·1
Prescribing: 3·1   range 1·8–4·0

Both of the above examples were very straightforward examples of consultations in which the diagnosis was not difficult and the problems presented by the diagnosis comparatively simple. It is also fair to observe that the patients were co-operative and provided all the information the doctor asked for.

Example 3

Let us now look at a much more difficult consultation in which the phases of the consultation are not in a simple sequence. The doctor involved in this consultation is the doctor who was involved in Example 1 in this chapter.

D. "Hello. Mrs K——?" (Seeking recognition.) "Come in and sit down." (Directing.) "What can I do for you?" (Broad opening.)

P. "Oh, I don't know. I'm just not feeling well at all."

D. "Do you have any pain?" (Direct question.)

P. "No, it's not pain. It's just that I can't sleep at all."

D. "Do you normally sleep well?" (Direct question.)

P. "Well, I haven't done for some months, you know."

D. "Is anything troubling you? Have you got a problem at home or something?" (Broad question, followed by a suggestion.)

P. "No, I don't think so. I just don't sleep and I am tired all day."

D. "You do look a bit run down." (Offering observation.)

P. "The kids are getting on my nerves and I shout at them in the evenings. My husband doesn't say much but I can see it upsets him."

D. "Now, you mustn't get too upset. We see a lot of this, you know." (Reassuring.) "Hop up there, will you? We'll have a little look at you just to check." (Directing.) "Now, I'm going to have a listen to your heart and chest." (Giving information.) "Take that coat off, will you?" (Directing.) "Good. Mmm. (Miscellaneous professional noises.) "Deep breath." (Directing.) "And again." (Directing.) "Mmm. Mmm. Yes. Mmm." (Miscellaneous professional noises.) "Have you got any tablets at all?" (Direct question.)

P. "Well, no. I haven't been to see a doctor in years." (1)

D. "Well, there's nothing wrong in there." (Giving information.) "You seem to be fairly healthy." (Reassuring.) "I think this is just a little something within yourself. I'll give you some tablets to take before you go to bed." (Summarising to close off.) (Giving information/directing.) (2)

P. "I've been having discharges for the last six weeks."

D. "Oh. Oh, you didn't tell me that." (Chastising.)

170

P. "Well, I've been having them for at least six weeks."

D. "Did they start at the same time as your sleeping problem?" (Placing events.)

P. "Well, they did and they didn't."

D. "I see. Well, we'd better have a look there as well." (A lot of instances of this sort of behaviour occur in consultations. It sounds like a way of seeking co-operation but, in fact, the real intention is to give the patient information about what is going to happen next. It is thus classified as "giving information".) "Will you go into the next room and get undressed? I'll be along in a minute." (Directing.)

   Three-minute gap not recorded.

D. "Have you ever had this before?" (Direct question.)

P. "Yes, I had it soon after I was married."

D. "I see. Did you see a doctor then?" (Direct question.)

P. "Yes."

D. "What did he diagnose?" (Direct question.)

P. "Well, he told me that it was due to the emotional strain of marriage. But that didn't make much sense, because I was very happy then."

D. "Did it stop?" (Closed question.)

P. "Well, it did for a while. Then it came back. That time he treated me for something to do with a gland or something."

D. "Let's see if there's anything in the notes." (Giving information.) "Ah, hum." (Miscellaneous professional noise.) "I see you were treated for a thyroid deficiency." (Concealed question.)

P. "That's it. But he stopped that after I went to see the specialist."

D. "What did he put you on then?" (Direct question.)

P. "Well, nothing. It went away, you see."

D. "Do you have any children?" (Direct question.)

P. "No. We've been trying for three years, but nothing happens."

D. "You haven't been for any tests or anything have you?" (Direct question.)

P. "Well, no. J—— won't go. He says he already has two from his first marriage and I'm . . . well, I don't know how to say it. . . . Well, I'm a bit worried about going."

D. "Well now, if it will put your mind at rest I'll arrange for you to have the tests—if you wish." (Pre-directional probing.) (3)

P. "Well, what does that mean? What will they do?"

D. "What do you mean, 'what will they do'?" (Clarifying.)

P. "Well, will I have to go into hospital?"

D. "No, not as a patient." (Answering patient question.) "But you will have to go to the hospital in the daytime to see the gynaecologist." (Giving information.)

P. "Will it hurt?"

D. "Not at all. It won't hurt a bit." (Reassuring.) "Now then, I'll fix it up and let you know when." (Giving information.) "It will be in about a fortnight, all right?" (Seeking patient ideas.) "I'll be in touch, okay?" (Summarising to close off.) "Right then, 'bye-bye." (Terminating.)

This consultation is more difficult to analyse because it has to start all over again (see (2)) when the patient volunteers a totally new symptom at the very point when the doctor thinks he has finished the consultation. Consequently, we have to treat this consultation as having two diagnostic phases and two prescriptive phases. Therefore, everything which follows (1) is prescriptive up to the point where the patient says:

"I've been having discharges for the last six weeks" when the consultation becomes diagnostic again.

The next decision he makes is at (3), when he is testing out the patient's willingness to undergo a series of tests.

Comparing his two prescriptive phases there is a marked difference. He is much more cautious in his second prescription because he changes his style of managing the patient. In the first prescriptive phase he gives a little reassurance, then gives information plus direction and closes. This style is very close to Style 2 (prescriptive). In his second prescriptive phase he tests a solution, deals with the patient's questions and then, finally, reassures and closes. This style is much closer to Style 4 (prescriptive). The actual scoring of this consultation is shown on the next pages.

His diagnostic score is thus 1·54 and his prescriptive score is 3·1.

The problem now facing the teacher is how to use this sort of information. If we look at the last example (Example 3), this case was used in a teaching situation to highlight certain points about the general nature of style. There were a number of criticisms which were essentially medical which are not the concern of this research. These apart, the following observations may be made.

Given the data which we presented on pages 162, 163 and the detailed lists (overleaf) the trainee can see for himself that he has a fairly consistent style of consulting which is slightly more flexible up to the point of diagnosis than it is after that point. In the consultation we have just quoted he did, however, find that his diagnostic style was inadequate because he only discovered a vital piece of information when he was on the point of prescribing a tranquillising drug. What clues are there in his style in this consultation which might give us an indication of where he made his mistake?

We cannot, in print, deal with his emphases or his mannerisms, but from the recording there was nothing in his opening which was other than cordial and friendly. The real clue lies in his response to the patient's first statement:

"I'm just not feeling well at all."

This can hardly be described as a helpful description of symptoms and the immediate response by the doctor is a wholly unsuccessful guess:

"Do you have any pain?"

The doctor tries to narrow down the possible response to an area where he could pursue an organic investigation. Instead of a reply in the affirmative all he got was a totally new lead about sleep. Again he counters with a direct question which leads him little further apart from raising the possibility that he might well be dealing with a non-organic problem.

The next mistake he makes is to offer a broad question and promptly close

172

CHECK LIST OF BEHAVIOURS WITH SCORE VALUES USED IN THE DIAGNOSTIC PHASES OF A CONSULTATION

Doctor Centered Behaviour	Score Value	Incidence 1st	Incidence 2nd		I x SV
Offering Self					
Relating to some previous experience					
Direct question	1½	111	111111		13½
Closed question	½		1		½
Self answering question (Rhetorical)					
Placing events in time or sequence or place	2		1		2
Correlational question					
Clarifying					
Doubting					
Chastising	1		1		1
Justifying other agencies					
Criticising other agencies					
Challenging					
Summarising to close off					
Repeating what patient said for affirmation					
Suggesting	1½	1			1½
Apologising					
Misc. Prof. noises	1½	11	1		4½
Directing	1½	11111	1		9
Giving information or opinion	2	1	11		6

Patient Centered Behaviour	Score Value	Incidence			I x SV
Giving or seeking recognition	1½	1			1½
Offering observation	3	1			3
Broad question	2½	11			5
Concealed question	3		1		3
Encouraging					
Reflecting					
Exploring					
Answering patient question					
Accepting patient ideas					
Using Patient ideas					
Offering of feeling					
Accepting feeling					
Using silence					
Summarising to open up					
Seeking patient ideas					
Reassuring	1	1			1
Indicating understanding					

Negative Behaviour	Score Value	Incidence			I x SV
Rejecting patient offers					
Reinforcing self position (justifying self)					
Denying patient					
Refusing patient ideas					
Evading patient questions					
Refusing to respond to feeling					
Not listening					
Confused noise					

Doctor Centered Behaviour	Score Value	Incidence 1st	Incidence 2nd	I x SV
Relating to some previous experience				
Directing	1½	1		1½
Clarifying	5½		1	5½
Doubting				
Chastising				
Justifying other agencies				
Criticising other agencies				
Challenging				
Summarising to close off	2	1	1	4
Repeating what patient said for affirmation				
Giving information or opinion	3	11	11	12
Advising				
Terminating (direct)	1		1	1
Suggesting				
Misc. Prof. noises				
Suggesting or accepting collaboration				

Patient Centered Behaviour	Score Value	Incidence		I x SV
Offering observation				
Broad question				
Encouraging				
Reflecting				
Exploring				
Answering patient question	4	1		4
Accepting patient ideas				
Using patient ideas				
Offering of feeling				
Accepting feeling				
Using silence				
Summarising to open up				
Seeking patient ideas	4½		1	4½
Reassuring	3	1	1	6
Terminating (indirect)				
Indicating understanding				
Pre-directional probing	4½		1	4½

Negative Behaviour	Score Value	Incidence		I x SV
Rejecting patient offers				
Reinforcing self position (justifying self)				
Denying Patient				
Refusing Patient ideas				
Evading patient questions				
Refusing to respond to feeling				
Not listening				
Confused noise				

174

CHECK LIST OF BEHAVIOURS WITH SCORE VALUES USED IN THE DIAGNOSTIC PHASES OF A CONSULTATION

Doctor Centered Behaviour	Score Value	Incidence	I x SV
Offering Self	1		
Relating to some previous experience	1½	卌 卌 卌 卌 卌	37½
Direct question	1½	卌 卌 卌 卌 卌 卌 卌 卌 III	64½
Closed question	½	卌 卌 卌 卌 卌 卌 卌 I	18
Self answering question (Rhetorical)	½	卌 卌 卌 卌	10
Placing events in time or sequence or place	2	卌 卌 卌 卌 卌 卌 卌 II	74
Correlational question	1½	卌 卌 卌 卌 卌 卌 II	48
Clarifying	3	卌 卌 II	36
Doubting	1½	卌 卌 卌 卌 II	33
Chastising	1	IIII	4
Justifying other agencies	1	II	2
Criticising other agencies	1	III	3
Challenging	2½	II	5
Summarising to close off	1	卌 卌 卌	15
Repeating what patient said for affirmation	2	卌 卌 卌 卌 III	46
Suggesting	1½	卌 卌 卌 卌 卌 卌 II	48
Apologising	1½	III	4½
Misc. Prof. noises	1½	卌 卌 卌 卌 卌 卌 卌 卌 IIII	66
Directing	1½	卌 卌 卌 卌 卌 卌 卌 卌 IIII	66
Giving information or opinion	2	卌 卌 卌 卌 卌 卌 卌 卌 卌 II	94

Patient Centered Behaviour	Score Value	Incidence	I x SV
Giving or seeking recognition	1½	卌 卌 卌 I	24
Offering observation	3	卌 卌 卌 卌 I	63
Broad question	2½	卌 卌 卌 卌 卌 卌 I	77½
Concealed question	3	卌 II	21
Encouraging	3	卌 卌 II	36
Reflecting	4		
Exploring	2½	I	2½
Answering patient question	2	卌 卌 卌 I	32
Accepting patient ideas	4	I	4
Using Patient ideas	3	I	3
Offering of feeling	2½		
Accepting feeling	4		
Using silence	4	III	12
Summarising to open up	3	I	3
Seeking patient ideas	4	IIII	16
Reassuring	1	卌 卌 卌 卌	20
Indicating understanding	2½	卌 卌 卌	37½

Negative Behaviour	Score Value	Incidence	I x SV
Rejecting patient offers	−1		
Reinforcing self position (justifying self)	−1		
Denying patient	−1		
Refusing patient ideas	−1		
Evading patient questions	−1		
Refusing to respond to feeling	−1		
Not listening	−2	卌 卌	−20
Confused noise	−1	卌 卌	−10

175

Doctor Centered Behaviour	Score Value	Incidence	I x SV
Relating to some previous experience	1½		
Directing	1½	ᴸᴴᴵ ᴸᴴᴵ ᴸᴴᴵ ᴸᴴᴵ ᴸᴴᴵ ᴸᴴᴵ III	42
Clarifying	5½	ᴸᴴᴵ ᴸᴴᴵ ᴸᴴᴵ ᴸᴴᴵ ᴸᴴᴵ ᴸᴴᴵ ᴸᴴᴵ	192½
Doubting	3		
Chastising	2	ᴸᴴᴵ ᴸᴴᴵ	20
Justifying other agencies	1	II	2
Criticising other agencies	1	III	3
Challenging	4		
Summarising to close off	2	ᴸᴴᴵ ᴸᴴᴵ ᴸᴴᴵ II	34
Repeating what patient said for affirmation	3	ᴸᴴᴵ ᴸᴴᴵ ᴸᴴᴵ	45
Giving information or opinion	3	ᴸᴴᴵ ᴸᴴᴵ ᴸᴴᴵ ᴸᴴᴵ ᴸᴴᴵ ᴸᴴᴵ I	93
Advising	3½	ᴸᴴᴵ ᴸᴴᴵ ᴸᴴᴵ ᴸᴴᴵ	70
Terminating (direct)	1	ᴸᴴᴵ ᴸᴴᴵ ᴸᴴᴵ	15
Suggesting	3	ᴸᴴᴵ ᴸᴴᴵ ᴸᴴᴵ IIII	57
Misc. Prof. noises	1	ᴸᴴᴵ ᴸᴴᴵ ᴸᴴᴵ ᴸᴴᴵ ᴸᴴᴵ ᴸᴴᴵ ᴸᴴᴵ II	37
Suggesting or accepting collaboration	4½	III	13½

Patient Centered Behaviour	Score Value	Incidence	I x SV
Offering observation	3½	I	3½
Broad question	3½	ᴸᴴᴵ ᴸᴴᴵ ᴸᴴᴵ ᴸᴴᴵ ᴸᴴᴵ ᴸᴴᴵ	105
Encouraging	5½	ᴸᴴᴵ ᴸᴴᴵ ᴸᴴᴵ ᴸᴴᴵ ᴸᴴᴵ I	143
Reflecting	6½		
Exploring	5½	ᴸᴴᴵ ᴸᴴᴵ ᴸᴴᴵ ᴸᴴᴵ I	115½
Answering patient question	4	ᴸᴴᴵ ᴸᴴᴵ ᴸᴴᴵ ᴸᴴᴵ II	88
Accepting patient ideas	6	ᴸᴴᴵ ᴸᴴᴵ	60
Using patient ideas	4½		
Offering of feeling	4½		
Accepting feeling	5		
Using silence	7	ᴸᴴᴵ II	49
Summarising to open up	5½		
Seeking patient ideas	4½	ᴸᴴᴵ ᴸᴴᴵ II	54
Reassuring	3	ᴸᴴᴵ ᴸᴴᴵ ᴸᴴᴵ ᴸᴴᴵ	60
Terminating (indirect)	4	ᴸᴴᴵ ᴸᴴᴵ	40
Indicating understanding	3	ᴸᴴᴵ ᴸᴴᴵ ᴸᴴᴵ	45
Pre-directional probing	4½	ᴸᴴᴵ ᴸᴴᴵ ᴸᴴᴵ ᴸᴴᴵ I	94½

Negative Behaviour	Score Value	Incidence	I x SV
Rejecting patient offers	−1	II	−2
Reinforcing self position (justifying self)	−1		
Denying Patient	−1	I	−1
Refusing Patient ideas	−1		
Evading patient questions	−1		
Refusing to respond to feeling	−1		
Not listening	−2		
Confused noise	−1	I	−1

176

it with another guess about domestic strain. He has to wait for the answer to this because the patient reiterates her symptoms. Then he drops his direct question and offers an observation on the way the patient looks to him:

"You do look a bit run down."

The change of strategy produces a totally different order of response because he suddenly gets part of the answer to the previous question about domestic strain. Inexplicably, he then stops this line of enquiry and proceeds as though he is fairly certain about his diagnosis. His short physical examination may then be seen as a fail-safe mechanism to remove any doubts he may have had. Then, having eliminated his doubts, he proceeds to close the consultation.

The comment we would make is that his questioning technique, very much Style 1, had the effect of limiting the patient to the sort of responses the doctor wanted to deal with. Having used a different strategy and having been rewarded with a much more valuable piece of information he then tried to deal with this situation as though he had made an organic diagnosis.

It was also pointed out to him during training that he was a little precipitate in assuming that his patient was in need of tranquillising. For his part he readily recognised that he had not let the patient talk sufficiently and had thus been in danger of over-simplifying the problem confronting him.

Training a trainee to cope with the problem of the patient who is slow to produce any real symptoms is not easy. It is possible to teach the trainee specific behaviours, as we indicated in the previous chapter. This particular trainee, however, shows a rather different problem. On the whole it would be unfair to say that he was particularly deficient in a wide range of behaviours. There are, admittedly, some gaps but he does have a reasonable range of what we have called "patient-centred behaviour".

The problem here is that his style is too limiting and needs to be enlarged. If this particular doctor could learn Style 3, for example, he would, arguably, be in a better position to cope with this sort of patient.

In Chapter 10 we gave an example of Style 3 (diagnostic) and a list of typical behaviours associated with that style. From this list it is evident that the trainee already has most of these behaviours (see page 107). The teaching task is thus to get the trainee to use more of these behaviours in a clear pattern and, if appropriate, to desist from asking as many direct questions based upon guess-work.

An introduction to the style could take the form of providing the doctor with the actual words used by the patient and requiring him, initially, to counter these statements with a behaviour which enables the patient to talk more openly or clarifies what she is talking about. The first part of the training for this particular doctor took this form:

Trainer: "I'm just not feeling well."

Doctor: "What do you mean by 'not feeling well'?"

Having successfully demonstrated a Style 3 behaviour he was then asked to produce more possible responses. A few are appended.

"I see. Go on."

"Mmm. Mmm."

"You are not feeling well?"

He was then asked to do the same for the following lead:

". . . It's just that I can't sleep at all,"

177

to which he produced the following:
"Tell me some more"
or
"What do you think about when you lie awake?"

This process can be repeated several times for as many inputs as the trainer cares to provide. Eventually, however, the trainee has to be confronted with a complete case so that he can try out his skills. As we have said in *Learning to Care*,[10] role-playing is a useful and safe device for this sort of learning because it gives the trainee freedom to experiment with new patterns of behaviour without risk. Eventually, he must be confronted with a live patient and here the trainer's discretion ought to be exercised to find a "suitable case".

A number of other issues arise out of this consultation which could well be the basis for discussion between trainer and trainee. There is contained within this consultation a very curious inconsistency. In the early part the patient says:

"The kids are getting on my nerves,"
but a few minutes later she tells the doctor that she has no children of her own which, indeed, leads him on to his final prescription.

There are also two possible leads about her relationship with her husband which do not cause any real response in the doctor, but may well have been significant if the patient had an emotional base for her condition.

In many of the consultations we have transcribed there are instances of patients producing apparently contradictory information, or of patients suggesting leads to doctors. The former problem is very easy to identify because it is easy to prove that, like all human beings, doctors are selective listeners. The problem with selective listening is that one usually selects on the basis of what one wants to hear. Listening is an essential part of any style and trainers should take account of the fact that trainees need to learn to listen.

As to the second problem of the suggested lead or the piece of inferred information there is no real way of analysing what the doctor cares to hear. Many of the doctors we have worked with refuse to accept inferred information and rarely wish to follow it up. It is not surprising that most of these doctors have shown that they also prefer to diagnose using Style 1.

Learning to use a completely new style is a problem we have not yet tackled. Growing styles from existing behaviours is not a really difficult task because no real new learning is involved. It simply requires a restructuring of skills already held by the trainee. We hope in the near future to start a project which will include such an objective within its programme.

Finally, we offer three cases in which the reader is invited to analyse and score the consultations and then to measure the style. In the diagnostic section there should be at least a difference of one complete style between each of the three, whilst in the prescribing style the difference should be greater.

Test Example No 1
D. "Good morning Mrs W——. Well now?"
P. "... I had a miscarriage at Christmas."
D. "Oh, I see, yes. How are you getting on?"
P. "Oh, all right."
D. "Have you had any period yet?"

178

P. "I've had two."
D. "Two, have you? When?"
P. "The third and twenty-seventh."
D. "And have you stopped losing now?"
P. "Yes."
D. "What were the periods like, were they heavy?"
P. "The first one was heavy, the second one was quite all right."
D. "Any trouble after the period?"
P. "No."
D. "No undue discharge?"
P. "No, not really."
D. "How long have you been married?"
P. "Two-and-a-half years."
D. "Have you any family?"
P. "No."
D. "How far had you gone when you had the miscarriage?"
P. "About eleven weeks."
D. "About eleven weeks. How did you feel about the miscarriage?"
P. "Oh, you know, it's the shock, it happened at Christmas and I went and...."
D. "Oh, my God."
P. "At seven o'clock. I think it's the shock more than anything."
D. "Yes, yes."
P. "I've only been out a few weeks. I just want a bottle."
D. "Yes."
P. "What do you think the odds are that it will happen again?"
D. "Oh, I don't know. Well, miscarriages are quite frequent I'm afraid...."
   Telephone.
D. "They are quite frequent. It's very difficult to explain why they occur, it's probably what they call a hormonal thing about the eighth and the twelfth week. Because you have one it isn't more likely that you'll have another, but they are quite frequent. I think it's about one in every forty pregnancies. So, really, the best thing is to forget it. It's probably as well to wait at least three months before you start with a pregnancy because you are more likely to miscarry if you start too soon with a pregnancy."
P. "Yes."
D. "Do you use any form of family planning or not?"
P. "At the moment we're using Durex."
D. "Yes. Everything's gone back all right so there's no reason why you shouldn't be all right."
P. "I'm still taking iron tablets."
D. "Yes."
P. "I don't know whether I need them or not."

179

D. "I'll just see about your blood. It was twenty-eighth December, yes?"

P. "I've put a lot of weight on."

D. "Have you?"

P. "I want to get rid of some."

D. "Well, try and get your weight down but I think as long as you get plenty of food you need not take any iron. All right?"

P. "Yes. Thank you very much."

D. "Goodbye."

Text Example No 2

D. "Come in, Mrs M——, sit down. Take your coat off . . . good, just lie on there. Any problems at all?"

P. "Not really, only very heavy pains down here. Not movement properly . . . and it's affecting my bowels as well."

D. "In what way?"

P. "Very loose, but you know, as though I'm running every two minutes, but it's just watery."

D. "Anyway, just lie on there. How long have you been before?"

P. "About three or four days now."

D. "Have you felt sick at all?"

P. "No, not really. Just a sort of upset stomach or, you know, pregnancy."

D. "Yes. Is your appetite normal?"

P. "Oh, I've had no appetite for ages with the heartburn. . . ."

D. "Well, I've been giving you tablets for heartburn, haven't I?"

P. "These pains seem to ease if I lie down and if I sit up. . . ."

D. "Well, you should be now thirty weeks."

P. "To my dates . . . well, you've got this eight weeks' difference and the thing is, it's next week or thereabouts . . . was wondering whether that had any affect on it, and really whether it would still affect me afterwards, because I had to go to the doctors and to the Family Planning Clinic, and one would say, 'Is she pregnant?' and one would say, 'No, you haven't got a "bulky womb" '. . . ."

D. "You see, a 'bulky' womb itself might be the explanation only, really, I don't think I've examined you when you're not pregnant, have I?"

P. "No, no."

D. "So, to give you that answer I would really have to give you an examination, and then we would know what your normal womb's like. It, maybe it's a bit soon and that could confuse the issue."

P. "In general, it's not just. . . ."

D. "Yes, in other words the starting-off point for your womb could be bigger than. . . ."

P. "It just worries me that the trouble I had before, whether it's going to re-occur."

D. "Well, I don't think you should worry unnecessarily, more often than not pregnancy does help these problems, but if you do come on afterwards we will have to look into it."

P. "You said when you examined me, like. . . ."

D. "Well, we will leave it at that and I'll see you in another fortnight, and don't worry, I am quite happy with the situation."

P. "Well, I'm due to see Dr—— on Tuesday at Crumpsall, so. . . ."

D. "Have you been taking your iron pills, now?"

P. "Yes, I've not been taking them these last few days and I wonder whether that might just be, you know. . . ."

D. "I'll give you some more."

P. "Can I have something for heartburn? Are there any other remedies other than those tablets you have given me?"

D. "Yes, there is."

P. "I don't know whether I'm immune to them or what, I've taken the full course of them instead of a fortnight, it's so bad, you know."

D. "There are some different ones. There you are. Two when necessary."

P. "Right."

D. "See you in a fortnight."

P. "I don't need anything to take with me to Crumpsall or anything like that?"

D. "No, I think he'll realise quite quickly the situation."

P. "See you Friday morning again, in a fortnight."

181

D. "Good morning, how are you today? Mrs J——, isn't it?"

P. "Yes, doctor."

D. "Well, what is it then?"

P. "Oh, I don't know what's up with me."

D. "Yes?"

P. "Well, I sit there with all the time in the world to do all the things I want to do and I . . . well . . . it's like this . . . I'm bored to tears. Then I get miserable . . . then I start to cry."

D. "Go on."

P. "Well, I'm there crying my eyes out for nothing at all. It's like being daft."

D. "Daft?"

P. "Well, it's only daft folk who do things like that. I think so, anyway."

D. "So you are crying for nothing and you think you are daft?"

P. "Well, don't you?"

D. "No, I don't. I've heard of people doing that before and I don't think they are daft. How long have you been married?"

P. "Eighteen months."

D. "Have you any children?"

P. "No. We decided to wait a bit. . . ."

D. "How long?"

P. "Maybe three years or so."

D. "What do you do in the way of work?"

P. "Oh, I don't work. He said that he wouldn't have me working once we were married."

D. "Your husband?"

P. "Yes. He's a bit old fashioned like that."

D. "I see. What did you do before you married?"

P. "Sales promotion. You know, going round to canteens and things giving away free cigarettes, or knocking on doors to get housewives to try some new rubbish or other."

D. "Did you enjoy that?"

P. "Oh, yes. I loved it, but you can't do that sort of thing when you're married."

D. "Why?"

P. "Well, you have to be away from home, sometimes for two or three days."

D. "Have you thought of going back to some other work?"

P. "Well, I have. But he won't have it. He says a man should look after his wife. God knows we've had that often enough."

D. "What do you mean by that?"

P. "Well, we have rows about it."

D. "Go on."

182

P. "Well, we had one this morning. I started to cry in bed before I got up. Then his breakfast was late and he was in a fair old mood."

D. "Is that why you came to me?"

P. "Well, yes. I'd like you to talk to him."

D. "You mean, you want me to ask your husband to let you go back to work?"

P. "Well, something like that."

D. "Will he come?"

P. "I'll try. Can I make an appointment for next Thursday?"

D. "You can. Do you think it will do any good?"

P. "Well, it's better than what's happening now."

D. "Right-ho. We'll do something like that then. I won't promise to ask him that question, though."

P. "Why?"

D. "That may not be the right thing to ask. Have you thought of that?"

P. "What?"

D. "Well, it may be deeper than just that."

P. "Well, all right. Let's see then."

D. "All right then, see you on Thursday. 'Bye-bye."

TEST EXAMPLE 1

CHECK LIST OF BEHAVIOURS WITH SCORE VALUES USED IN THE DIAGNOSTIC PHASES OF A CONSULTATION

Doctor Centered Behaviour	Score Value	Incidence	I x SV
Offering Self			
Relating to some previous experience			
Direct question			
Closed question			
Self answering question (Rhetorical)			
Placing events in time or sequence or place			
Correlational question			
Clarifying			
Doubting			
Chastising			
Justifying other agencies			
Criticising other agencies			
Challenging			
Summarising to close off			
Repeating what patient said for affirmation			
Suggesting			
Apologising			
Misc. Prof. noises			
Directing			
Giving information or opinion			

Patient Centered Behaviour	Score Value	Incidence	I x SV
Giving or seeking recognition			
Offering observation			
Broad question			
Concealed question			
Encouraging			
Reflecting			
Exploring			
Answering patient question			
Accepting patient ideas			
Using Patient ideas			
Offering of feeling			
Accepting feeling			
Using silence			
Summarising to open up			
Seeking patient ideas			
Reassuring			
Indicating understanding			

Negative Behaviour	Score Value	Incidence	I x SV
Rejecting patient offers			
Reinforcing self position (justifying self)			
Denying patient			
Refusing patient ideas			
Evading patient questions			
Refusing to respond to feeling			
Not listening			
Confused noise			

TEST EXAMPLE 1

PRESCRIBING BEHAVIOURS CHECK LIST OF VALUES FOR STYLE CALCULATION

Doctor Centered Behaviour	Score Value	Incidence	I x SV
Relating to some previous experience			
Directing			
Clarifying			
Doubting			
Chastising			
Justifying other agencies			
Criticising other agencies			
Challenging			
Summarising to close off			
Repeating what patient said for affirmation			
Giving information or opinion			
Advising			
Terminating (direct)			
Suggesting			
Misc. Prof. noises			
Suggesting or accepting collaboration			

Patient Centered Behaviour	Score Value	Incidence	I x SV
Offering observation			
Broad question			
Encouraging			
Reflecting			
Exploring			
Answering patient question			
Accepting patient ideas			
Using patient ideas			
Offering of feeling			
Accepting feeling			
Using silence			
Summarising to open up			
Seeking patient ideas			
Reassuring			
Terminating (indirect)			
Indicating understanding			
Pre-directional probing			

Negative Behaviour	Score Value	Incidence	I x SV
Rejecting patient offers			
Reinforcing self position (justifying self)			
Denying Patient			
Refusing Patient ideas			
Evading patient questions			
Refusing to respond to feeling			
Not listening			
Confused noise			

TEST EXAMPLE 2

CHECK LIST OF BEHAVIOURS WITH SCORE VALUES USED IN THE DIAGNOSTIC PHASES OF A CONSULTATION

Doctor Centered Behaviour	Score Value	Incidence	I x SV
Offering Self			
Relating to some previous experience			
Direct question			
Closed question			
Self answering question (Rhetorical)			
Placing events in time or sequence or place			
Correlational question			
Clarifying			
Doubting			
Chastising			
Justifying other agencies			
Criticising other agencies			
Challenging			
Summarising to close off			
Repeating what patient said for affirmation			
Suggesting			
Apologising			
Misc. Prof. noises			
Directing			
Giving information or opinion			

Patient Centered Behaviour	Score Value	Incidence	I x SV
Giving or seeking recognition			
Offering observation			
Broad question			
Concealed question			
Encouraging			
Reflecting			
Exploring			
Answering patient question			
Accepting patient ideas			
Using Patient ideas			
Offering of feeling			
Accepting feeling			
Using silence			
Summarising to open up			
Seeking patient ideas			
Reassuring			
Indicating understanding			

Negative Behaviour	Score Value	Incidence	I x SV
Rejecting patient offers			
Reinforcing self position (justifying self)			
Denying patient			
Refusing patient ideas			
Evading patient questions			
Refusing to respond to feeling			
Not listening			
Confused noise			

TEST EXAMPLE 2

PRESCRIBING BEHAVIOURS CHECK LIST OF VALUES FOR STYLE CALCULATION

Doctor Centered Behaviour	Score Value	Incidence	I x SV
Relating to some previous experience			
Directing			
Clarifying			
Doubting			
Chastising			
Justifying other agencies			
Criticising other agencies			
Challenging			
Summarising to close off			
Repeating what patient said for affirmation			
Giving information or opinion			
Advising			
Terminating (direct)			
Suggesting			
Misc. Prof. noises			
Suggesting or accepting collaboration			

Patient Centered Behaviour	Score Value	Incidence	I x SV
Offering observation			
Broad question			
Encouraging			
Reflecting			
Exploring			
Answering patient question			
Accepting patient ideas			
Using patient ideas			
Offering of feeling			
Accepting feeling			
Using silence			
Summarising to open up			
Seeking patient ideas			
Reassuring			
Terminating (indirect)			
Indicating understanding			
Pre-directional probing			

Negative Behaviour	Score Value	Incidence	I x SV
Rejecting patient offers			
Reinforcing self position (justifying self)			
Denying Patient			
Refusing Patient ideas			
Evading patient questions			
Refusing to respond to feeling			
Not listening			
Confused noise			

TEST EXAMPLE 3

CHECK LIST OF BEHAVIOURS WITH SCORE VALUES USED IN THE DIAGNOSTIC PHASES OF A CONSULTATION

Doctor Centered Behaviour	Score Value	Incidence	I x SV
Offering Self			
Relating to some previous experience			
Direct question			
Closed question			
Self answering question (Rhetorical)			
Placing events in time or sequence or place			
Correlational question			
Clarifying			
Doubting			
Chastising			
Justifying other agencies			
Criticising other agencies			
Challenging			
Summarising to close off			
Repeating what patient said for affirmation			
Suggesting			
Apologising			
Misc. Prof. noises			
Directing			
Giving information or opinion			

Patient Centered Behaviour	Score Value	Incidence	I x SV
Giving or seeking recognition			
Offering observation			
Broad question			
Concealed question			
Encouraging			
Reflecting			
Exploring			
Answering patient question			
Accepting patient ideas			
Using Patient ideas			
Offering of feeling			
Accepting feeling			
Using silence			
Summarising to open up			
Seeking patient ideas			
Reassuring			
Indicating understanding			

Negative Behaviour	Score Value	Incidence	I x SV
Rejecting patient offers			
Reinforcing self position (justifying self)			
Denying patient			
Refusing patient ideas			
Evading patient questions			
Refusing to respond to feeling			
Not listening			
Confused noise			

TEST EXAMPLE 3

PRESCRIBING BEHAVIOURS CHECK LIST OF VALUES FOR STYLE CALCULATION

Doctor Centered Behaviour	Score Value	Incidence	I x SV
Relating to some previous experience			
Directing			
Clarifying			
Doubting			
Chastising			
Justifying other agencies			
Criticising other agencies			
Challenging			
Summarising to close off			
Repeating what patient said for affirmation			
Giving information or opinion			
Advising			
Terminating (direct)			
Suggesting			
Misc. Prof. noises			
Suggesting or accepting collaboration			

Patient Centered Behaviour	Score Value	Incidence	I x SV
Offering observation			
Broad question			
Encouraging			
Reflecting			
Exploring			
Answering patient question			
Accepting patient ideas			
Using patient ideas			
Offering of feeling			
Accepting feeling			
Using silence			
Summarising to open up			
Seeking patient ideas			
Reassuring			
Terminating (indirect)			
Indicating understanding			
Pre-directional probing			

Negative Behaviour	Score Value	Incidence	I x SV
Rejecting patient offers			
Reinforcing self position (justifying self)			
Denying Patient			
Refusing Patient ideas			
Evading patient questions			
Refusing to respond to feeling			
Not listening			
Confused noise			

CONCLUSIONS

Three-and-a-half years' examination of doctors and their behaviours have enabled us to draw some conclusions. The first of these is that it is possible to analyse a complex human activity such as the doctor/patient consultation, and from that analysis derive information which should be beneficial to the process of doctor training. This conclusion of researchers has been supported by the feedback received from many of the doctors who have attended the experimental programmes based on our findings.

The possible applications of this information are also becoming clear. We believe it to be unwise to consider placing any training in behaviours in the first two/three years of medical school, because the learner would be acquiring interactive skills prior to any real comprehension of the tasks which form the basis for their exhibition. During the three years in hospital there are few opportunities to consider the development of such learning.

Rationally, the learning of such skills should form part of the experience a doctor will have once his chosen apprenticeship in the field of general practice has begun. Once someone has made the decision to be a GP, then is the time for his training to become more specific.

At present the training of GPs is as varied as the number of institutions which offer the training. This in itself is no bad thing, because it allows the development of different schools of thought and different approaches to the problems. In any human activity there will never be a set of perfect prescriptive answers to all the situations thrown up by that activity. Answers, however, usually depend upon the questions which are asked, and here there is considerable room to doubt much of what is done in the name of GP training.

When one attends conferences of GP trainers it is difficult to discover what the trainers themselves think they are doing. There are long debates about the viability, desirability, and even the validity of methods of training, in the complete absence of any real debate about why a particular method has been chosen, and what objectives it is presumed to serve.

On balance, one comes to the conclusion that a great deal of the training of GPs is based upon a confused pattern of objectives. To some extent *The Future General Practitioner*[3] has offered a range of learning goals and objectives, but despite the wide sale of this work the confusion still exists. Certain propositions need to be clear about GP training. In the first place it takes place immediately after the completion of a long period of intensive undergraduate training. It should be unnecessary, therefore, that the programme should concern itself with matters which have already been dealt with in the course of a normal medical curriculum. If, however, there is a particular general practice emphasis in the medical content, if that emphasis is proven to be of special importance to general practice, then it is necessary that this emphasis be exhibited.

Secondly, there is a concealed purpose in such training which ought to be made clear. One of the purposes of such training is to enable a would-be GP to decide whether or not general practice is what he wishes to spend the rest of his life doing. The training period is thus a filtering process as well.

Thirdly, there are vital propositions to make about standards. The only purpose of any training is to raise and/or accelerate the achievement of standards. The level of performance of any particular GP is not simply measured in terms of his diagnostic and prescriptive skills. His task is to create long-term human relationships within which he will practise his unique form of medicine. Creating long-term human relationships comes easily to some and not so easily to others. It is difficult to imagine how high standards of general practice can be achieved without the efficient creation of these relationships. To a great extent what we have been examining in this study has been some aspects of a human relationship which lend themselves to a degree of quantification. We would not wish to offer our approach to the consultation as a panacea for the problems of those who find it difficult to form effective human relationships. It could be that general practice is not for such. Where, however, the research might help, is in the presentation of alternative ways of improving skills which are already there.

It will be observed that we have refrained from any attempt to define the perfect consultation. We do so because no such thing exists. As this is a bi-focal approach, a coming together of behavioural science and general practice, we have often concluded that what is good to one party may well be disaster to the other. Equally, a doctor's doctor is not the same thing as the patient's doctor. What we have learned, however, is that the consultation is a complicated mixture of the discipline we call medicine and the effective utilisation of behavioural skills. We may, therefore, talk about consultations which are more effective and consultations which are less effective. Yet the final arbiter of what we have set out to do will be the GP himself. We do not set out to sell him a package of instant skills and behavioural tricks which will remove all difficulties, all the warts and wrinkles from his style, or from that of his trainee. What we are offering here is a sort of camera with which one may take a picture of one aspect of a doctor's performance, even a self-portrait. Given such a picture, the doctor concerned is then left to decide whether or not he is satisfied with what he sees. We also believe that what we have uncovered has a not insignificant bearing upon the content of the training of the GP of the future.

In the course of this research we have learned much about issues which lie completely outside the scope of the work itself. We have been concerned simply to understand some aspects of the behaviour of the GP in his consulting-room. Yet some of the insights we have obtained do have a bearing upon areas of medical education which have implications beyond the training of GPs.

What is apparent is the fact that doctors, like any other professional group, are both a product and a prisoner of the training system which has produced them. Over the last 20 years it is true that medical education has changed considerably, but in the main these changes have reflected the development of one new scientific approach to medicine at the expense of another, perhaps currently unfashionable, area. The main function of medical education has, quite rightly, maintained an emphasis upon the prevention and cure of organic disease. We have rarely been in a position to assess the effectiveness of any of the diagnoses offered by those doctors who have provided us with tapes. When we have worked with groups of doctors and they have considered each other's consultations, arguments about the actual diagnosis have been few and usually of the same kind. The debate has almost invariably been over whether the doctor concerned has accepted the initial offer of symptoms and has failed to detect a not so obvious underlying psychological and/or psychosomatic disorder.

To expect doctors to make an accurate diagnosis every time is a nonsense.

191

The consultation is, after all, a human activity and as such is prone to a degree of error. That some consultations do end with a bad or inaccurate diagnosis is inevitably true. That there are doctors who are inefficient and lazy is true. But the reverse is also true. There are brilliant and life-saving diagnoses and there are more doctors who are thoroughly efficient and anything but lazy. It is probably also true that poor doctors make good copy for the media, whilst good doctors, like good news, are bad copy.

Many of the failures well-published by the media are rarely as simple as we are led to believe. For years we have had debates and arguments over the two ethically difficult areas of birth control and abortion. Much bad publicity has centred on doctors who will have nothing to do with either. The problem arises when a patient demands these "services" as of right. It is all very well for legislators to create laws which produce a system in which these services may be sought and provided. It is quite another matter to force a doctor to do anything which fundamentally transgresses his personal system of belief.

For us these issues are not the failings of general practice. We all, doctors or not, commit two sorts of sins—one of omission and one of commission. One sin which we commit is to treat the prescription of various drugs and the prescription for a life style as tasks of an equal order of magnitude (qv). We have already written on the insensitive way in which some doctors give advice to some of their patients. This we believe springs from a very real lack of comprehension and understanding of the lives of their patients. At a very simple level, taking two pills three times daily is not of the same order of activity as "taking things easy for a while", whatever that may mean. In many ways Cronin's two doctors, Finlay and Cameron, are one man—the ideal doctor. One practises careful medicine but is really concerned to care for the life style of his patients. The other is more able at the spectacular diagnosis and the efficacious modern remedy. Together the two of them represent one ideal doctor.

Doctors do, on occasions, give advice to patients which it is quite impossible for the patient to follow. Just as a bad teacher will "teach all day without anyone learning a thing" so the bad doctor will doctor all day whilst the patient refuses or is unable to cure himself.

The other sin is the sin of omission. Many doctors feel hopeless when faced with a "sick" patient who has nothing organic wrong with him. The incidence of psychosomatic and psychosocial disorder is either on the increase or we are becoming more able to detect its presence. Many of the doctors we have worked with have been most defensive on this issue. Some refuse to believe such illness exists while some who recognise it claim that it falls outside their own responsibility.

These beliefs do still still exist, yet G. M. Carstairs[20] wrote and broadcast the following in 1962:

"Perhaps nowhere in contemporary society can be seen such clear evidence of the persistence of magical thinking as in the doctor's willingness to be persuaded (well, half persuaded) that the drug houses have the newly discovered elixir of life. In recent years extravagant hopes have been centred upon the psychotropic drugs, drugs which will relieve agitation and depression, and others which calm the turmoil of the acutely deranged. These drugs are often effective, if only for a time; but they have been used so intemperately that we still know remarkably little about their scope and limitations and their possible dangers; and yet they are being prescribed today in their millions. I do not wish to deny the help these drugs have brought to many seriously ill patients, but only to point out that when they are taken to relieve the emotional distress caused by problems of living they are merely anodyne, and offer no lasting solution."

What Carstairs wrote then is as true today. While the causes of this aspect of doctors' behaviour are complex, many can be traced back to the training, or lack of it, received in medical school. It took many years for the study of psychology to be included in the medical curriculum, and even today it remains one of the Cinderella subjects. Clinical psychology is, however, only one kind of insight into man's condition. Carstairs appeared to draw much from his reading of the classical sociologist, Durkheim. Sociology provides yet other windows into the condition of man, and it is probable that the coming together of psychology and sociology in the discipline now known as social psychology will provide new and crucial windows through which to view and understand the roots of psychosocial disorder.

Without the broad perspective on mankind provided by what are now called the "behavioural sciences" it is not surprising that doctors fail to come to terms with such illnesses. One cannot search for something unless one knows what one is looking for and where to look for it. We must stress, by repetition, that our statements on what we have observed reflect much more on his training than ever they do on the doctor.

We have also observed that there are some aspects of patient behaviour which are equally curious.

On tape we have heard doctors being asked advice on major issues for which they have in no way been trained. To what extent is a doctor able to give advice, other than medical, to a 62-year-old teacher who is contemplating retiring three years before his expected retirement date? Equally, is a doctor the right person to give advice to a patient about whether or not she should remain in a state of marriage to a man she detests? Can a doctor give adequate advice to a parent on the "right" way to bring up children? Most of these issues are as remote from his previous curriculum as are the relative merits of various gas cookers—yet we have one doctor being asked the latter question.

As our society is becoming increasingly secular, it is often the doctor who is being asked to assume the role traditionally played by priests. It is doubtful if doctors have asked for this role, although quite a few have honestly attempted to fulfil it, formally untrained though they may be. If patients keep on asking doctors these questions then presumably doctors will come under increasing pressure to answer them. There may well be another side to Michael Balint's "apostolic function", namely the "willing disciples syndrome" in which doctors are seen by patients as the essential oracle to be consulted at all possible times.

There is a type of patient who will come to see a doctor regularly, every week perhaps, in order to have someone to talk to. We do not know whether such a patient comes because of conditioning by the medical profession, or whether the patient comes because there is no one else to talk to. The fact remains that patients do come and consult doctors on issues which are often non-medical. We may therefore ask, should not medical education respond to this demand—or should it quietly ignore it in the hope that the patient and the problem will go away?

We have also learned things about patients in this study which can, any day, justify separate pieces of research, which we would be most interested to undertake. We feel that Balint's propositions have been clearly supported in a number of the samples we have offered, and, with the reservations noted above about the "willing disciple syndrome", much of what Balint had to say is good advice for the medical profession.

We have on occasions had cause to speculate about the degree to which patients use doctors for reasons other than medical reasons. Doctors are asked to answer questions which might have taxed even Solomon in all his wisdom. We have already offered some of these, but below are a few examples of some of the other odd questions which have been put to unsuspecting GPs.

"Do you think I ought to go to Greece for a holiday this year?"

"Did you hear about Mrs X? Those twins—they are not her husband's you know. They've got blue eyes. They can't have blue eyes from him can they?"

"Do you think I ought to let him have his mother come to stay with us next year?"

"If I live with him before I get married what do you think my mother will say?"

It is interesting to speculate why people go to doctors to seek this sort of advice. Clearly the doctor must occupy an important role in their lives. We accept that many patients use questions like this to approach obliquely the reason for their being there, but there still must exist a substantial number of "genuine enquiries".

The dangers of this are, of course, the dangers of the self-fulfilling fantasy. If people keep on asking a doctor to answer such questions the doctor will eventually run the risk of having fantasies about his role in life. As long as the questions keep on being asked the fantasy will be more likely to be reinforced to the point of its becoming a reality rather than being extinguished. We hope that the results of this research will be useful in helping doctors to cope with patients.

What we have described is but Phase I of a longer study. We now hope to commence Phase II. Here we will seek to compare the performances of trainees of doctors who have learnt to use our methods of analysing their own behaviours and styles, with trainees of doctors who have not had such training themselves. Can self-analysis of verbal behaviours go some way to the achievement of greater effectiveness for patients and greater "job satisfaction" for the doctor? We believe that it can.

REFERENCES

1. Byrne, P. S., Harris, C. M. and Long, B. E. L. (1976). "Teaching the teachers." *Medical Education, 10,* 189–192; Harris, C. M., Long, B. E. L. and Byrne, P. S. "A teaching methods course in Manchester for general practitioner teachers." *Medical Education, 10,* 198–204; Long, B. E. L., Harris, C. M. and Byrne, P. S. "A method of teaching counselling." *Medical Education, 10,* 198–204.

2. Browne, K. and Freeling, P. (1976). *The Doctor-Patient Relationship.* 2nd edition. London and Edinburgh: Churchill Livingstone.

3. Royal College of General Practitioners (1972). *The Future General Practitioner. Learning and Teaching.* London: British Medical Journal.

4. Spence, J. (1960). *The Purpose and Practice of Medicine.* London: Oxford University Press.

5. Taylor, S. (1954). *Good General Practice:* London: Oxford University Press.

6. Flanders, N. A. (1960). *Interaction Analysis in the Classroom: a Manual for Observers.* Ann Arbor: University of Michigan Press.

7. Bales, R. F. (1950). *Interaction Process Analysis.* Massachusetts: Addison-Wesley.

8. Hays, J. S. and Larson, K. H. (1963). *Interacting with Patients.* New York: Macmillan.

9. Scott, R., Anderson, J. A. D. and Cartwright, A. (1960). "Just what the doctor ordered: an analysis of General Practice", *British Medical Journal, 2,* 293–299.

10. Byrne, P. S. and Long, B. E. L. (1973). *Learning to care: person to person.* Edinburgh and London: Churchill Livingstone.

11. Berne, E. (1966). *Games People Play. The Psychology of Human Relationships.* London: Andre Deutsch.

12. Balint, M. (1964). *The Doctor, his Patient and the Illness.* London: Pitman.

13. Bales, R. F. and Gerbrands, H. (1948). "The interaction recorder: an apparatus and check-list for sequential content analysis of social interaction." *Human Relations, 1,* 456–463.

14. Flanders, N. A. (1963). *Helping Teachers Change Their Behaviour.* Ann Arbor: University of Michigan Press.

15. Rackham, W., Honey, B. and Morgan, R. G. T. (1971). *Interactive Skills.* Wellens.

16. Sanhammer, N., Hays, J. S. and Larson, K. H. (1962). *Interacting with Patients.* W.H.O. Working Group Report.

17. Rogers, C. (1951). *Client Centered Therapy.* Boston: Houghton Mifflin.

18. Hodson, M. (1967). *Doctors and Patients. A Relationship Examined.* London: Hodder and Stoughton.

19. Fulton, A. E. (1970). "The measurement of speaker credibility." *Journal of Communication, 20,* 270–279.

20. Carstairs, G. M. (1963). *This Island Now.* London: Hogarth Press.

Printed in England for Her Majesty's Stationery Office
by The Campfield Press, St. Albans

(22145) Dd 290468 K.16. 10/76.